Improving the Menopause Experience
Through Nutrition and Lifestyle

of related interest

Black and Menopausal
Intimate Stories of Navigating the Change
Edited by Yansie Rolston and Yvonne Christie
Foreword by Iya Rev. DeShannon Barnes-Bowens, M.S.
ISBN 978 1 83997 379 6
eISBN 978 1 83997 380 2

The Personalized Nutrition Guide to Menopause
Christine Bailey
ISBN 978 1 80501 144 6
eISBN 978 1 80501 145 3

Menopause Yoga
A Holistic Guide to Supporting Women on their Menopause Journey
Petra Coveney
Foreword by Dr Louise Newson
ISBN 978 1 78775 889 6
eISBN 978 1 78775 890 2

Women's Health Aromatherapy
A Clinically Evidence-Based Guide for Nurses, Midwives, Doulas and Therapists
Pam Conrad
ISBN 978 1 84819 425 0
eISBN 978 0 85701 378 1

Maintaining Strength, Mobility and Optimal
Strength Health Through the Life Stages
A Guide for Women's Health and Fitness Professionals
Dr Jen Wilson and Dr Athalie Redwood-Mills
ISBN 978 1 80501 339 6
eISBN 978 1 80501 340 2

Improving the Menopause Experience Through Nutrition and Lifestyle

THE TRIANGLE OF HORMONAL HEALTH

Claire Snowdon-Darling and Laura Knowles

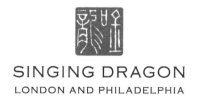

SINGING DRAGON

LONDON AND PHILADELPHIA

First published in Great Britain in 2025 by Singing Dragon,
an imprint of Jessica Kingsley Publishers
Part of John Murray Press

I

Copyright © Claire Snowdon-Darling and Laura Knowles 2025

The right of Claire Snowdon-Darling and Laura Knowles to be
identified as the Author of the Work has been asserted by them in
accordance with the Copyright, Designs and Patents Act 1988.

All rights reserved. No part of this publication may be reproduced, stored
in a retrieval system, or transmitted, in any form or by any means without
the prior written permission of the publisher, nor be otherwise circulated
in any form of binding or cover other than that in which it is published and
without a similar condition being imposed on the subsequent purchaser.

The information contained in this book is not intended to replace the services
of trained medical professionals or to be a substitute for medical advice. You
are advised to consult a doctor on any matters relating to your health, and in
particular on any matters that may require diagnosis or medical attention.

A CIP catalogue record for this title is available from the
British Library and the Library of Congress

ISBN 978 1 80501 187 3
eISBN 978 1 80501 188 0

Printed and bound in Great Britain by CPI Group UK Ltd

Jessica Kingsley Publishers' policy is to use papers that are natural, renewable
and recyclable products and made from wood grown in sustainable
forests. The logging and manufacturing processes are expected to conform
to the environmental regulations of the country of origin.

Singing Dragon
Carmelite House
50 Victoria Embankment
London EC4Y 0DZ

www.singingdragon.com

John Murray Press
Part of Hodder & Stoughton Limited
An Hachette UK Company

The authorised representative in the EEA is Hachette Ireland,
8 Castlecourt Centre, Dublin 15, D15 XTP3, Ireland (email: info@hbgi.ie)

For the women whose stories and struggle inspired us to find the answers.

Contents

PREFACE 9

Part One: What is happening during menopause?

1. Introduction. 13

2. Today's menopause situation 21

3. What is the Triangle of Hormonal Health? 35

4. Blood sugar hormones 41

5. Stress hormones. 61

6. Sex hormones 75

7. Digestive function 97

8. Immune function. 117

9. Putting the Triangle of Hormonal Health together 129

Part Two: How can I make my menopause better?

10. Menopause is a gift – no, really.... 133

11. How to reduce your stress(ors) 139

12. Hormone replacement therapy (HRT). 167

13. What is the best diet during menopause? 181

14. Navigating symptoms with a staged approach 199

15. Conclusion. 229

16. Next steps and resources 231

17. Frequently Asked Questions 237

    THANKS AND ACKNOWLEDGEMENTS. 243

    REFERENCES 245

Preface

In late 2021, a 15-year-old came into Claire's clinic. She had been first struggling with some skin issues but despite having had a first period, they hadn't continued. She had been to the doctor but had been told that because she wasn't 16, they wouldn't do any blood tests. She had been offered the contraceptive pill and the usual skin meds such as antibiotics and Roaccutane. Her mum, who is educated in nutrition and complementary approaches, wanted to avoid this approach. Claire spent some time discussing the connection between her hormones, the lack of bleeds and her skin, and they set about a course of action of removing some obvious foods that could be causing an issue and supporting the young woman's body to make the hormones it needed to. The young woman complied entirely with the dietary tweaks, and her skin improved, but the bleeds didn't return. Understanding that it was essential to get these hormones kick-started as the menstrual cycle is a key indicator of a woman's health (and fertility), Claire asked them to request a blood test from the GP. Despite being denied on a few occasions, the mother and daughter fought to be heard and finally had a blood test which showed that the young woman had very low levels of progesterone, which could be treated with natural progesterone, but this was not offered because it's not how the medical model works. They finally found a private GP who would issue the progesterone. Six months of "textbook" periods ensued, but when the prescription ran out, her bleeds stopped again, so Claire explained it was now time to fight hard to find a hormone doctor who would do tests to find out why the issue was happening and who would support her with natural progesterone.

Another young woman (21 years old) had come off the contraceptive pill after being on it for a few years and her bleeds hadn't returned. The doctor had told her not to worry until she wanted to have children. After battling the GP, they gave her a blood test, but because they didn't test for her progesterone levels, the test results came back as "normal", and she was diagnosed with polycystic ovary syndrome (post-pill PCOS is common) – again, the treatment for this is to be offered the contraceptive pill.

— 9 —

Claire advised the woman to pay privately for a blood test (which is often prohibitively expensive) and the results showed that she too had untraceable amounts of progesterone. She then had to work with a private Harley Street doctor at more expense to be prescribed natural progesterone as the GP wasn't allowed to give it to her.

These young women were essentially walking into an early menopause without intervention, and yet the current medical approach meant doctors must refuse the treatment that is freely available, has minimal side effects and can fix the issue that these women are dealing with.

We have heard, on repeat, hundreds of shocking stories of perimenopausal women being refused full blood tests, not offered the correct treatment and dismissed because this isn't important or life-threatening. But the symptoms these women are experiencing are life-affecting. Working with menopause has meant listening to women feeling helpless, unheard, dismissed, mocked, and commonly misdiagnosed and mis-medicated.

All these stories combined made us realize there is a systemic failure in the management of women's hormones – not just during menopause but throughout our entire lives – and it has got to the point where we couldn't sit back and allow this to continue without trying to change it.

This is why we have written this book. It's why we teach practitioners across the world to be able to support women going through these issues, why we run our clinic and why we work tirelessly to change the current system. It feels like a David versus Goliath fight, but we can't allow another generation of women to experience being failed. For every woman who becomes empowered to get the right treatment and to feel better, it makes the battle worthwhile.

With so much love,
Claire and Laura

— PART ONE —

What is happening during menopause?

— CHAPTER 1 —

Introduction

Millions of women are struggling with a very challenging menopause. They have tried everything and feel broken, lost, scared, and confused. They have been bombarded with conflicting information and don't know where to turn. Doctors are often unable to help them due to a lack of understanding and training. Although celebrities are bringing the topic of menopause into the mainstream media, the information they are promoting is the same one-size-fits-all medical approach, with no explanation as to why this doesn't work for a lot of women. When the standard approach doesn't work, it is common for women to feel dismissed and mistreated.

The truth is that for many of these women, their issues started long before perimenopause. Their health history is often littered with red flags and warning signs of a body that is struggling: irritable bowel syndrome (IBS), headaches, period anomalies, fertility issues, anxiety, weight problems, and burnout are all trivialized as "normal". But they aren't normal; they are signs of an impending hormonal storm at perimenopause that can be life-affecting.

These women often find that because of these underlying issues, they can't tolerate HRT, or it is ineffective, they are unable to sleep, they have developed allergies, rashes, horrendous anxiety, or depression, and the hot flushes and vaginal dryness are overwhelming.

The medical profession is in free fall. Women are struggling to see their GPs, and when they do, they are commonly prescribed a myriad of other medications such as antidepressants or sleeping tablets rather than a form of HRT that could help them. There has been an overwhelming request for natural HRT, and in 2023 we saw a supply issue that caused huge disruption. But for many women, this approach also isn't working.

Health coaches supporting these women are equally confused. They are often on their own journey with menopause, and although many are researching or looking to train in this subject, they commonly state that information is sparse, conflicting, or baseless.

We have spent years watching women trying the latest fad, only to end up more unwell.

Who are we?

"We are Claire Snowdon-Darling and Laura Knowles. Best friends since we met in 2000, health seekers since 2004, and business partners since 2010.

Professionally, we are highly qualified kinesiologists, nutritionists, emotional coaches, and teachers. We have both been in private clinical practice since 2007 and have worked with thousands of women.

Having taught for other colleges, we set up the College of Functional Wellness in 2019 as a route to training excellent health coaches to work with menopause, wellness, Functional Kinesiology, and emotional coaching. Our college is now international and accredited with the most prestigious authorities in the world, and we train hundreds of students every year. Our work is regularly featured in the press, and we are often speaking at events and seminars, in business and menopause groups across the country.

We live, sleep, eat, and breathe figuring out the hormone issues at the root cause of conditions.

Personally, we have both struggled with life-affecting symptoms since our 20s, which catapulted us on to the path of self-discovery and research – primarily to heal our own issues but also to help others.

Our stories seem very different, but the similarities have been what caused us to dive deeply into research.

Claire experienced general health issues in early life such as weight problems, chronic migraines, and irritable bowel syndrome. However, in 2004 she experienced major birth trauma and blood loss while giving birth to her daughter, Mya. This resulted in postpartum psychosis, postnatal depression, post-traumatic stress disorder (PTSD), and chronic fatigue syndrome. Her 15-year struggle with these conditions finally led to a diagnosis of primary ovarian failure in 2016, and she has since been experiencing an extremely challenging menopause, where none of the standard solutions work and she has had to battle to regain her quality of life.

However, Claire's struggle meant that she left no stone unturned in her quest for health, and this has resulted in the creation of the Triangle of Hormonal Health in 2015. She has been in remission from chronic fatigue syndrome since 2021.

Laura has had a 25-year struggle with life-affecting irritable bowel syndrome and chronic skin issues. Through her teens, Laura was on repeated antibiotics for tonsillitis and hospitalized several times from its severity. At the age of 20, she had her tonsils removed, which was meant to be a solution, and woke up with a skin condition that was diagnosed as the autoimmune disease guttate psoriasis. Despite having seen doctor after doctor and specialist after specialist, and trying every remedy and cream known to man, this condition stubbornly stayed put. The official diagnosis has been questioned numerous times by numerous experts as it doesn't behave like psoriasis at all. She spent years in her 20s on different types of contraceptive pills, which compounded the hormone, digestive, and immune issues. Her skin and gut issues were compounded by crippling anxiety and fertility issues; through her research, it became apparent that there was a connection between all these symptoms.

We have both experienced being let down, dismissed, misdiagnosed, overprescribed, and lied to by both doctors and complementary medical practitioners, and we have dedicated our lives to researching the root causes of issues to break through the health myths and to provide empowering, helpful information to women to ensure they can make informed decisions that take them back to health.

That is why we are writing this book: to give coaches and women the information they need to make sense of what is happening and to give them guidance on what to do to feel better.

In this book, we are going to bring you the latest scientific, nutritional research and demystify it to provide jargon-free explanations about what is happening during the menopause transition. We will show you how different hormonal interplays often link together to create a storm of symptoms. Our gift is taking complicated information and breaking it down to make it interesting and understandable.

We are passionate about educating women to understand their body and to make informed choices around diet and lifestyle changes, and empowering them to be able to have the conversations with their doctors about the right approach and HRT for them, should they need it.

The strategies provided in this book, created through years of clinical practice and research, offer you the information needed for yourself or for others to make informed decisions on healthcare and reclaim full vitality and wellbeing during the transition into the next stage of life.

One of the main criticisms we hear from people is "you aren't doctors". That is correct: we are not doctors – we are coaches. We have some of the same information at our disposal as doctors, but we have an entirely different approach to how we use that information.

It is coaches, not doctors, who have the time and information to support women with their health issues. Coaches are at the front line, the same as the medics, but we have resources that doctors could only dream of – engaged clients who are willing to work on changing habits, time to offer effective coaching – and we can respond quickly to new information. The NHS system has overlooked this precious commodity for too long and historically labelled us as charlatans. However, we are now seeing coaches working alongside progressive and pioneering doctors who are pushing back against the entrenched system, and we are making waves of change in healthcare.

Women's health is complicated, and issues with women's health generally don't fit the medical system where an issue is dealt with where it manifests.

Historically, women have been significantly under-represented in medical research. It was as recently as 1993 that US legislation was passed to ensure that women are represented in all clinical research.[1] And in the UK, it was only in 2020 that guidance was issued on sex and gender representation.[2] There was an incorrect assumption by researchers that there were no significant differences between men and women regarding medication response, and therefore no need to study women separately. There was also the inconvenience of having to adjust for women's fluctuating hormone levels during her monthly cycle, and concern over reproductive effects.

Many of the common medications prescribed today were developed and trialled before the 1990s and therefore were only tested on and designed for men.

Another complication with the medical approach is its segmented view. For example, if you have gut pain, you will be referred to a gastroenterologist; if you have unexplained migraines, you will see a neurologist; and if you have joint issues, you will see a rheumatologist. This all sounds logical, except that when you understand how inflammation works systemically, you understand that the condition manifesting in a specific place often has nothing to do with the cause of that condition. But the medical model isn't concerned with "why" a condition is there; its focus is to stop it in its tracks using appropriate intervention such as surgery or medication. While that is all well and good, it is all too common for symptoms to appear in a new place once we've stopped them somewhere else.

The medical model is reductionist, and the gaps caused by this myopic view become all too apparent during the menopause transition if a woman is struggling because of her past health issues. The "cut it out or medicate it" approach can make things ten times worse for women with hormone imbalances or autoimmune conditions when the body is already in crisis.

Medicine has its place, but what rarely happens is a clear explanation of the risk versus reward with medications. There is always a biochemical change that happens when we take medication, and part of the decision-making process should be "Is the health improvement I may experience from this drug worth the risk of change in function or side effects that could result?" But women are not given the opportunity to explore this question and are often told that a medication is a solution to their health issues. When you look at a woman's whole health history, you can often see clearly that dietary and lifestyle issues are at play, and by educating and supporting a woman how to change them, you can negate the requirement for the medications prescribed.[3]

The Hippocratic oath states "first do no harm", but what we will explore is that by focusing on synthetic hormones, often due to financial pressure, without looking at the root cause of conditions, and by applying medications and often unnecessary surgery, women *are* being harmed, every single minute of every single day. We have seen hundreds and hundreds of women who are very, very damaged by this approach, and it is genuinely heart-breaking.

The science is out there to access the root cause of a condition, but the medical system, with its budget constraints and lack of resource, doesn't allow for it to be at the fore of the service women receive.

We want to be clear; it is not doctors that we have an issue with. Doctors are often highly intelligent, hard-working professionals who are dedicated to helping people. But the system they find themselves in is broken. Not just the NHS (and thank you, UK, for having a free medical service that people can access) but all the medical healthcare systems have become about profit, surgery, and pharmaceuticals, and not a whole-health approach.

If we ever get hit by a bus, we will be incredibly grateful to receive the NHS care and attention, and Claire is open about how she has needed support from the medical approach many times in her health journey. It has a place; it's just that it doesn't work when we are talking about hormones, menopause, digestion, or the immune system.

While many still consider coaches or complementary therapists as inferior to the medical model, it is the fact that we are not in a "system" that makes coaches so useful. It is our differences from the medical model that mean we can call upon a variety of information and disciplines to find the right approach for the client in front of us.

We have dedicated our careers to training excellent coaches, highly qualified to be able to support women to make the best choices for their health, be that an offering from the medical profession, the naturopathic profession, or a combination of both.

But the issue with coaches is that the complementary health world is unregulated, and so the education that coaches receive can be incredibly varied. This is compounded by the fact that the internet is full of conflicting and often outdated, misleading, and, in some cases, dangerous information.

Until recently, the phrase "nutritional science" was a misnomer. There was little science and a lot of guesswork, but the leaps and bounds that have been made in the past 20 years are staggering and have proven that pretty much everything we thought we knew about nutrition and how the human body works was wrong.

The joy of working in our industry is that progress is fast, plentiful, and rapidly changing. We look forward to building on the knowledge we have in the future. For us, researching health and hormones doesn't stop.

IMPROVING THE MENOPAUSE EXPERIENCE THROUGH NUTRITION AND LIFESTYLE

But for now, this is what we offer you with this book – the most up-to-date information and research on perimenopause and menopause as it stands in 2024. We offer you the bridge between the science and the naturopathic, with simple-to-understand explanations of what is happening in the body in the run-up to and during the menopause transition. We hope it will be full of "aha" moments that can help you make decisions that take you back to wellness.

How to use this book

The information in this book is layered. It has been written in a certain order for a reason, so it is important to read it in that order. This has been tried and tested hundreds of times because it's how our courses work. You need the information from one chapter to understand what is truly happening in the next chapter. Please trust us on this and follow the pathway as it was designed to be followed.

Part One is all the information you will need to understand what's happening to the body in the menopause transition, and it may start to feel like a bleak outlook, but don't worry: Part Two is where we look at all the solutions.

This book is going to be talking about hormones. A lot.

Hormones are mostly talked about in relation to the menstrual cycle, but our whole body runs on hormones. They are our chemical messages; they are produced to send and receive information between all parts of the body and the brain. Everything from realizing you need the loo to feeling tired is a message that has been delivered by a hormone. This system is intricate and complex, and it is also completely overlooked.

We are going to be deep-diving into what we call the "five pillars of health". These pillars focus on how hormone destabilization wreaks havoc in our body. These pillars are blood sugar hormones, stress hormones, sex hormones, digestive function, and immune function. Understanding them will give you the "whole health" picture. Some of these may sound unrelated to menopause, but all will become clear by the time you've finished reading this. You will see how it all fits together.

At the end of the book, we have plenty of resources for you to access to help you embed the changes we recommend. This is a deeply empowering and educational journey, and we hope you love the unfolding as much as we have loved discovering this pathway.

Thank you for allowing us to join you on your path. We truly find it an honour to have the opportunity to be part of your journey to wellness. If it helps you understand what is happening, *please* pass on the knowledge, to your friends, family, and clients. Women are great at supporting each other. This woman-to-woman exchange of information is how we have always educated ourselves historically, and it's also how we have risen up and fought against injustice. The general approach to women's health is brutal, dangerous, and wrong, and it needs us to rise up and fight for change. We cannot allow the next generation of women to go through what we are going through. If shining a light on this approach can change the future for our daughters, nieces, granddaughters, and the girls in our community, then we must do what we can. This revolution only requires that we stop putting our health into the hands of others and learn for ourselves what is going on in our bodies. Then we can finally demand the right treatment and support.

But that can only happen when we feel well and energized, so let's get started.

Note: While we use the term woman a lot throughout the book we want to acknowledge that the menopause affects a wide range of people, such as those who are non-binary and trans men.

— CHAPTER 2 —

Today's menopause situation

Menopause is hitting the headlines and has become a buzz word for the first time. On the one hand, it's great that we are talking about it more openly and removing the stigma and shame attached with this hormonal transition. On the other hand, information that doesn't fit the mainstream narrative feels limited. The few options given to women tend to be medicalized, and women who don't feel magically "better" with the blanket approaches often end up feeling more lost, hopeless, and alone. As if they have somehow failed at something.

There is a wide range of celebrity influencers now driving the discussion: Davina McCall, Lisa Snowdon, Mariella Frostrup, Michelle Obama, Penny Lancaster, and Gwyneth Paltrow to name a few. Each of them has a slightly different message – for example, Davina McCall is campaigning for free hormone replacement therapy (HRT), while Lisa Snowdon is campaigning for education and awareness around the topic, and Gwyneth Paltrow is encouraging women to understand more about perimenopause.

It is all excellent progress; however, millions of women are falling through the gaps because often these messages promote a one-size-fits-all approach to HRT (often synthetic HRT) and usually reflect the issues that the celebrity struggled with personally.

In the UK, we have celebrity doctors whose expensive private clinics promote high-dose oestrogen therapy and often have little aftercare for clients who experience fallout from this approach. We have had many clients who have been badly advised to be gung-ho with their hormone therapy and feel awful because of it. They are then told it can't be the treatment as "no one else has had an issue". Bearing in mind we know at least a dozen women who have had this experience, we know this isn't true.

The issue with the media and the influencers and the celebrity doctors comes down to one common factor: they aren't addressing the underlying conditions that lead to women struggling in the first place. If women have gut issues, they might not be able to absorb their HRT, and they can often feel awful. If women have an overstimulated immune system or a history that includes fatigue disorders, it can be challenging for them to sail through menopause naturally, and many of the mainstream options for HRT often trigger reactions.

These women aren't in the minority, however. Having spoken to and worked with literally thousands of menopausal women in a variety of countries, we hear these same stories repeatedly, and it's time for women to access the information that they need to be able to navigate this transition.

The menopause experience is a wide and varied spectrum. Some women get through the characteristic "year without a period" with no symptoms bar a few warm flushes. Others are so unwell that they feel the only option is death.

The Office for National Statistics recorded that among women, age-specified suicide was highest between the ages of 45 to 49.[1] Similarly in Australia, the data echoes this information with the two peaks of age-specified suicide being 45–49 and 50–54,[2] and the US showed similar data of age-specified suicide highest being in those aged 45–60.[3]

In clinic, we see first-hand how common it is for women to talk about "not wanting to be here any more" because they feel so awful, and they don't want to live this way.

In 2020, the world locked down because of the COVID-19 pandemic. As therapists, we couldn't work in our clinics, and we were mindful that many clients were unable to access support during this challenging time. We decided to create an online Hormone Assessor – basically, a health quiz that gave women guidance on where to start making changes to their diet and lifestyle to help them navigate their way back to health.

The data we've collected since then has been astonishing.

Out of 2112 people who completed the Hormone Assessor, 98 per cent were women. Of those women, 69 per cent were perimenopausal, 86 per cent were struggling to maintain a healthy weight, a staggering 97 per cent were stressed and always busy, while 94 per cent said they were exhausted with not enough energy, and 93 per cent were anxious or overwhelmed.

In addition, 93 per cent were eating sugary foods regularly and 88 per cent had digestive issues.

Although it's a small batch of data, it's compelling and terrifying to see the state of women's bodies at the time of life when they need to navigate the menopause transition.

What is going on?

The women going through menopause today are the first generation of women who weren't just told that they could have it all but were actively encouraged to have it all. Get good grades at school, carve out a career, get married, have a perfectly kept house whose interiors wouldn't look out of place in *Homes & Gardens*, have children and be a model parent, but don't let your career slide, keep up with your social life and always give a perfect dinner party, rollerblade during your period, starve yourself to maintain a size-10 body, don't age, make sure to put Botox and filler in your face and colour your hair, be sexually adventurous and super sexy, look glamorous, and don't forget to keep your sense of humour. Pep yourself up with caffeine and sugar, eat low-fat foods, be in calorie restriction, and rush around all day to make sure that nothing falls by the wayside.

It's too much. And the result is that the women who have tried to achieve it all have hit menopause and keeled over.

In the 1950s, the housewives had their issues (one of which was systemic boredom that led to high levels of alcohol and tranquilizer abuse), but their daily patterns allowed for periods of rest and recovery.

It was common for a woman in this era to get her husband and children out of the door and sit down to have her breakfast in peace with a magazine or the radio on in the background.

It was uncommon for households to own cars, and certainly not two cars, so there was unlikely to be a "school run", followed by the relentless list of errands that today's women have.

You find us a woman who has a break in her day to have a cup of tea and listen to the radio, because we've never met one. These days, if we find ourselves with a gap, we fill it with a job from the endless "to-do list" or by scrolling through social media. There is no actual rest. And, for most of the women we've worked with, the idea of "self-care" and taking time out leads to a landslide of guilt.

As much as we are committed feminists and believe in equality, the truth is that a woman's body wasn't designed to cope with this much sustained pressure. Unlike men, our hormones work cyclically, which means our energy is also cyclical. We were meant to rest during our bleed, but that isn't possible with today's high-pressured lifestyles. In fact, historically, when we were forced out of the village to live in a communal tent during our bleed, tribe elders would cook the food and look after the children while the women who were bleeding rested. This practice still exists in parts of the world, and while there is still often the stigma of being "unclean" to overcome in these societies, the concept of rest during a menstrual cycle is a welcome one.

Throughout our lives, therefore, we put a significant amount of stress on our bodies and hormones, and by the time we get to perimenopause, our body can't handle this major transition. We like to use the word "bandwidth". In these days of a constant requirement of connectivity to the internet, we know too well what happens when too many people try to get online at the same time. The Wi-Fi can't cope. It slows down or stops working altogether. It's the same for our bodies. Our body only has capacity to deal with a certain amount of stress. If there is too much stress, we run out of bandwidth and our system falls over.

An example of this would be spending years eating foods we know aren't good for us. We have got into the habit of grabbing food on the go, snacking on sugary foods, propping ourselves up on coffee. We might have low-level symptoms such as headaches or a bit of a sluggish bowel or a persistent muffin top, but nothing that is too challenging. Our body is "buffering" the issues that this kind of diet is causing.

But then the stress ramps up. We take on a new job or we have another baby, and we are using up even more bandwidth.

This is often the case before we even hit perimenopause, when our hormones naturally become unstable. Perimenopause takes up vast quantities of bandwidth, and if we've used too much previously, we won't physically be able to manage, and symptom after symptom will start to appear. Modern women have literally run out of bandwidth by the time they hit menopause.

What is menopause?

There are a lot of words bandied around about menopause and they can be confusing.

Pre-menopause is when we are in our fertile years. We are experiencing a monthly cycle.

Perimenopause is when we start to experience some early menopause symptoms. As discussed in Chapter 1, these can be incredibly subtle and start much earlier than we expect them to begin. It is common to experience perimenopause symptoms up to ten years before the actual menopause commences.

Menopause is the time that our periods stop or are beginning to become destabilized. This can go on for a few years.

Post-menopause is when we have had 12 consecutive months without a bleed. In the case of early menopause (before the age of 40), 24 consecutive months are required without a bleed. If we bleed in this time, we are still either in late perimenopause or going through the menopause, but it's hard to tell and there isn't a way to find out accurately. It's a "wait and see" situation, and it's very common to get ten months in or more and then have a bleed and be back to square one (Claire got to 364 days without a bleed, then started bleeding again monthly!).

The phrase "menopause" is commonly used as an umbrella term for the whole period that spans the perimenopause to post-menopause transition. Even though women can spend up to 20 years going on the journey from perimenopause, through menopause, and into post-menopause, we still don't talk about the process openly. Doctors often miss the symptoms of perimenopause, and women can suffer with the fallout for years before blood tests will show this is what is happening.

What are the symptoms of menopause?

The NHS website states that there are 34 symptoms of menopause.[4] Some websites say 39.

A search online will yield the list of symptoms below, and many of these are well known and to be expected during menopause. It becomes a little trickier if you are experiencing these symptoms in your mid- to late 30 as doctors assume it's too early for menopause; women can be given a diagnosis of another condition and often prescribed medication, often incorrectly, such as antidepressants or beta blockers. These often do nothing to fix the issue as the issue really needs hormone stabilization.

1.	Hot flushes	16.	Sense of taste issues
2.	Night sweats	17.	Itchiness
3.	Vaginal dryness	18.	Tingling extremities
4.	Decreased sex drive	19.	Electric sensations
5.	Breast soreness	20.	Burning mouth
6.	Irregular periods	21.	Digestion changes
7.	Bloating	22.	Muscle aches
8.	Headaches	23.	Disrupted sleep
9.	Mood swings	24.	Thinning hair
10.	Fatigue	25.	Osteoporosis
11.	Depression	26.	Irregular heartbeat
12.	Anxiety	27.	Weight gain
13.	Irritability	28.	Memory lapses
14.	Panic disorder	29.	Concentration lapses
15.	Joint pain	30.	Brittle nails

31. Incontinence

32. Dizziness

33. Allergies

34. Body odour changes

It's a lot to have thrown at you! This list of symptoms is well documented and, in some cases, sounds quite benign, but it doesn't consider the spectrum of intensity of these symptoms that women experience. "Itchiness" doesn't sum up the feeling of a thousand ants being trapped under your skin 24/7, or a scalp so itchy that you are waking in the night with your fingernails embedded in your head.

The list doesn't come close to painting the full picture of what can happen during perimenopause and there are some symptoms that are often overlooked, such as:

- sudden onset intolerance to food you ate regularly – commonly, these are shellfish and fermented foods such as Prosecco

- digestive issues including heartburn

- fluid retention and blood pressure changes

- sudden knee or hip pain with no obvious trigger

- life-limiting anxiety and a feeling of doom or such an absence of joy and "colour" in the world that it feels pointless to continue

- life-limiting fatigue disorders onsetting in your 30s without an obvious trigger

- being so forgetful you don't remember to turn the hob off

- losing words and names, often to the point that it compromises your work

- sequencing issues and doing strange things like leaving your car keys in the fridge

- bleeding so heavily that you are flooding through sanitary products regularly and can't leave the house

- spotting every few weeks

- being so intolerant of people, noises, movement, and light that you become insular and retreat socially.

Faced with a myriad of these symptoms, which are often completely out of character for the individual, the question that is commonly asked is "Am I going mad?" It can really feel that way, and looking at this list, it's not hard to see why, if unsupported and untreated, suicidal ideation is common. In clinic, we have seen repeatedly that women usually burst into tears with relief when they hear that these symptoms are common, and they aren't alone.

According to the website NHS.inform, the average age for menopause in the UK is 45–55 years. Basic maths would therefore tell us that many, many women fall outside of this age bracket, and in clinic we have certainly seen a lot of women experiencing early perimenopause symptoms in their mid-to late 30s.

These symptoms may not be enough for a woman to seek help from her GP, but they are enough to cause issues with her quality of life, relationships, and physical and mental health. If she were to seek help, perimenopause would largely be dismissed as a cause, due to her younger age.

When women start to develop strange symptoms, even if they are in their 30s, and especially if they have had children in their mid- to late 30s, it is a *major* red flag that their hormones are starting to fluctuate. Having the right support at this stage can save a lot of problems later.

These symptoms could include:

- sleep issues

- sudden unusual anxiety around daily tasks such as driving

- confidence issues which weren't there before

- an increase in food intolerances

- weight gain

- increased fatigue

- being noticeably snappier than before

- period changes such as bleeds becoming heavier, lighter, or more irregular.

Because these symptoms could be a variety of other conditions, it is common for women to be dismissed by their GP or sent to the wrong specialist for further investigation. For example, it is common for women to see a gynaecologist when experiencing cycle irregularities, not a hormone specialist (endocrinologist). While a gynaecologist will probably order some blood tests, it is unlikely they would order the same tests as a doctor with an in-depth knowledge of hormone issues.

Being told that "nothing is wrong" and that "test results are normal" is commonplace. This was Claire's experience for 12 years. The average time it takes for a woman to get a diagnosis of endometriosis is eight years. This is because if a condition isn't easy to see in a test, or the wrong tests were performed, the woman is dismissed or sent back to the GP and must start from square one again.

The truth is that medical tests are surprisingly limited when it comes to hormones. Blood tests can tell us if the hormones are present and if they are in the right amount, but the test doesn't give any information about how the hormones are being used by the body. An example would be blood testing for the stress hormone called cortisol. A blood test will simply show if there is cortisol in the blood and how much.

A urine or saliva test takes samples at different times of day. This test can analyse how much cortisol is released and when and how the body is using it. These are called "functional tests". They aren't the standard tests used by the medical model and are limited to the realm of functional and complementary medicine. They are therefore paid for privately and can be very expensive, which makes them inaccessible to many people.

The NHS also now will not test a woman's hormones if she is over the age of 45, which seems ridiculous when this is the exact time we need to have our hormones tested. The policy is to hand out HRT but without finding out which HRT is the right one for each individual or which of our hormones are depleted. This means we can overload women with too many hormones too early on in their perimenopause, or flood their body with synthetic hormones that can wreak havoc, especially on a system that was already struggling. This creates a cascade of other symptoms, often worse than the symptoms the woman had before she went on HRT. These could include depression, anxiety, blood pressure anomalies, heartburn, digestive issues, weight gain, palpitations, insomnia, being tired but wired, and nausea. And, at worst, this could increase the risk of stroke or cancer.

Many women experiencing these symptoms will be offered medication, and it is common for a woman to have a long list of pills as she goes through menopause, such as antidepressants, statins, beta blockers, sedatives, prescription painkillers, and stomach acid suppressants.

However, as we will explore in later chapters, many of these issues are linked to how our body is handling stress as well as the depletion in hormones during menopause. While for some women this medication is essential and life-saving, for many others, it is mis-prescribed because the doctors often don't have the time or training to spot that the issue is due to a hormone imbalance, and if they do, they don't have the resources to investigate the situation thoroughly.

It is hard to believe that GPs are not trained in menopause, but a shocking number are not. It seems essential – after all, half of us will go through this transition – but in January 2023 the British government rejected a recommendation by the House of Commons Women and Equalities Commission for GPs to take mandatory training in menopause, meaning that it is a lottery as to whether or not the GP you are talking to is able to support you effectively at a time when you need as much help as you can get.

We were at a medical conference in spring 2023 where a speaker asked how many delegates had been to medical school. Approximately 300 hands went up in the air. He then asked the delegates to leave their hands in the air if they had been trained in menopause. Only about a dozen remained.

This is a problem because the current guidelines for working with menopause are, in our view, missing the big picture, and we need well-trained doctors to understand the nuances happening as our hormones start to fluctuate.

The current practice stems from recently updated guidelines for working with menopause called the 2023 Practitioner's Toolkit for Managing Menopause;[5] originally developed in 2014, this approach is endorsed by the International Menopause Society and the British Menopause Society.

These guidelines state that:

- No blood tests should be offered for women over the age of 45. This is because it should be simple to diagnose a woman of this age with menopause if she has had no bleed for 12 months and offer HRT. However, as we will explore in this book, the symptoms and issues associated with perimenopause are commonly happening many years before periods become irregular or stop altogether, and as women are getting to 45, we are commonly in the most unstable part of our menopause, where we have too much of some hormones and not enough of others. By not testing what is happening with a woman's hormones, doctors are blindly offering her a full dose of HRT, which she may not need or be able to tolerate and which often makes her feel much, much worse. In our view, this guideline is stopping millions of women from getting the support they need and deserve.

- Hormone testing may be used for women aged 40–45 and for women without bleeds with subtle or fluctuating symptoms (such as mood change). This test will be a single observation of the hormones FSH (follicle-stimulating hormone) and oestrogen but *not* progesterone or testosterone. As we will show you in later chapters, progesterone is the most important hormone to test with these subtle symptoms and in these early stages of perimenopause. This guideline leaves women feeling lost and helpless when commonly their test results come back as "normal" when they feel anything but.

- Hormone tests are required to diagnose a condition which presents as early menopause called primary ovarian insufficiency/premature

— 29 —

ovarian failure (POI/POF), but this testing often misses out progesterone, and many women can go for years and years with this being missed. (Claire experienced a decade of having this condition missed due to the lack of testing progesterone.)

- If women have had a full hysterectomy, they should be prescribed oestrogen only instead of oestrogen and progesterone (unless they have had a history of endometriosis or have had a sub-total hysterectomy). As we will show, this is a major oversight as progesterone is hugely implicated in a woman's mood (and her ability to sleep).

- Synthetic progesterone (progestin) is essential for endometrial protection for women who still have a uterus. We absolutely, resolutely disagree with this, and as we will be showing you, synthetic progesterone has very little, if any, benefit whatsoever, and, in fact, can be a major cause of ill health in women. Natural progesterone is a different story as you will learn. This guideline is based on shaky evidence at best, and we truly believe that it is damaging women.

- Breast cancer is a contraindication to the use of HRT. While we agree that hormonal breast cancers are a contraindication to HRT, many women are being excluded from being offered life-changing hormones because of a blanket ban.

- The prescription of individually formulated and compounded hormone preparations is not recommended. This is due to the lack of available research, but, in our view, bearing in mind how many women cannot tolerate the standard HRT route, it seems remiss to continue to avoid doing the research.

- There is presently no evidence-based indication for testosterone therapy for women. Although it is acknowledged that it may improve sexual desire, there is no evidence. As we will show, testosterone does a lot more than increase our libido, and so again we say, go and do the research.

- Natural progesterone has been shown to be safer than synthetic progesterone (progestin) with regard to breast cancer risk in observational studies. This highly important point is in the small print and not in the recommendations. This leads us to question why synthetic progesterone is being touted.

- If menopausal symptoms persist on the highest dose of oral therapy, there is little point increasing beyond the recommended upper dose, and it is advised to switch to a non-oral alternative. If symptoms persist, then testing must be carried out to check if a woman is absorbing the dose. This again is a hugely overlooked recommendation and is in absolute contrast to the trend for offering women more and more oestrogen without any exploration as to why their HRT isn't working for them.

The current medical approach endorsed by NICE (the National Institute for Health and Care Excellence, which creates evidence-based recommendations for healthcare in England) was published in 2015. It mirrors the new toolkit described above, except that NICE allows for HRT to be used to treat depression and low mood. But again, it is often too much of the wrong hormone at the wrong time that is being offered, and the progesterone is commonly in the form of a synthetic hormone, which isn't beneficial.

This is the problem we are facing. The guidelines don't reflect what women are dealing with, and even when the guidelines state that further exploration should happen, it usually doesn't.

There are a small number of people trying to highlight these issues with the guidelines including journalists, prominent functional doctors, and researchers (and us), but we are so far not being heard. We are determined to create a sea change in the current approach.

We've mentioned early menopause, so let's explore this subject further.

Early menopause

We can have an early menopause for a variety of reasons, including:

- chemical or surgical menopause as a side effect of having a total hysterectomy or oophorectomy

- premature ovarian failure/primary ovarian insufficiency (POF/POI)

- primary pituitary dysfunction.

In our experience, chemical and surgical menopause or menopause caused by POF can be difficult to navigate.

In the case of chemical or surgical menopause, there was usually a condition in the body that led to the decision to have surgery, such as cancer, fibroids, or endometriosis.

Women are often unable to have HRT if the original issues were due to hormonal imbalances, but this leaves women floundering without a lifeline and feeling horrendous.

With POF, the diagnosis of early menopause feels reductionist as the

— 31 —

journey a woman had to endure even to get to the point of diagnosis can include a lot of life affecting symptoms such as fatigue disorders (e.g, chronic fatigue, ME, or fibromyalgia), and mental health issues such as depression or overwhelming anxiety. It can take a decade of being told that there is "nothing wrong" before getting this diagnosis.

The cause of the body going into early menopause is usually overlooked by the medical model, and doctors are often dismissive once the diagnosis has been found.

Once found, the response is to issue HRT, but often, in these cases, women are going through a complex array of hormonal imbalances, and simply replacing "lost" hormones isn't enough. In many cases, the HRT can't be tolerated due to the underlying issues such as a history of gut dysbiosis and IBS or migraines. The root cause still needs to be dealt with or the symptoms will continue, but now these will be accompanied by the menopause symptoms.

All too often, women fall through the cracks in the overstretched health system and aren't offered counselling, support, or guidance on being told that they are now infertile and have been thrust into premature ageing with all the life-limiting symptoms this brings, such as osteoporosis and heart issues.

It is also important to note that even with the complex issues at play with early menopause, once diagnosed, a woman won't get any financial support from health insurers because this is a "natural transition". Except, in this case, it isn't. Something has gone wrong, and whatever it was that went wrong will now be sidelined because the result is menopause. If women want to get to the root cause of what is making them feel so unwell, they will be expected to pay, and this can cost many, many thousands of pounds.

Primary pituitary failure can be caused by the use the contraceptive pill or because a woman's bleed didn't start properly when she was in puberty. In these instances, the messaging to and from the pituitary gland stops working effectively and the menstrual cycle doesn't happen.

Often this condition goes undiagnosed for years as in early puberty, the medical model won't explore causes for the lack of a bleed; often, by the time it is explored, it's too late. The medical response for this is to give synthetic hormones, but this doesn't fix the issue, just masks it.

For women coming off the pill, they won't have any investigations done by medical practitioners for at least 18 months, by which time it is often too late for the pituitary gland to start working properly again. This cause of early menopause is surprisingly common and yet, to our knowledge, women aren't advised that the pill could cause early menopause, and therefore infertility, when they are in the throes of making the decision about which form of contraception is right for them.

In our clinics, however, we have seen an astonishing amount of perimenopause symptoms in younger women.

Young women today are having to cope with huge amounts of stress, and throughout the book we will be exploring what is happening in the body and why symptoms happen. While the focus of this book is perimenopause to post-menopause, it is important to note that the same hormone stressors are happening for younger women. It is these stressors and the hormone fallout caused that are contributing to the rising number of issues and conditions we see in the world today – from diabetes to PCOS, endometriosis, and fertility problems. The root causes are the same for these conditions as they are for a woman navigating a challenging menopause – a lack of bandwidth leading to hormonal fallout and subsequent symptoms.

HRT can be a major problem in today's menopause. The first HRT options created all centred around oestrogen replacement, and the medical model still focuses on the importance of oestrogen and often overlooks the importance of progesterone. Often, though, women who have complex medical histories leading up to a challenging menopause have warning signs of a progesterone deficiency as far back as their teens. In fact, perimenopause is a "progesterone deficiency" condition, as we will explore. Giving women more oestrogen during this time often exacerbates their symptoms.

But that is only part of the problem. Unless her GP has had training in menopause, it is likely that a woman will be given HRT options that contain synthetic progesterone. As we will be discovering later, this synthetic progesterone can cause a lot of issues and even stop your body's own progesterone creation process.

There are natural progesterone options available, but they are often not prescribed because they are more expensive, the GP often doesn't know about them, and, more disturbingly, medical practices are financially incentivized to promote specific options. Specifically in women's health, the Mirena coil is a commonly prescribed option that financially benefits the doctor's practice. The physical and emotional fallout that women can experience from a Mirena coil is well documented online. How can we trust that the doctor prescribing it is doing so in our best interest if we know that there is financial reward and targets to be met?

The science behind it is also entirely flawed, as we will discuss in Chapter 12.

The constraints of time and resources in the medical system mean that women are often pushed into a one-size-fits-all approach, which doesn't always work, and, again, women are dismissed when they question if their prescription is working.

On top of the physical issues, there are the emotional aspects of going through menopause that can be challenging. Menopause and ageing still hold a lot of shame and stigma for women. The common themes are around a loss of self-worth, striving for eternal youth, grieving our lost youth, and struggling with the changes in our body.

But, despite all of this, there is hope. So much hope.

Even if we are struggling with our menopause, this major life transition has great gifts to offer us. It can force us into radical self-care and creating healthy boundaries, and it might be the first time in our life when we learn to put ourselves first.

In our experience, when a woman can understand what is happening in her body, she is able to make changes to her diet and lifestyle to reduce the stress in her system and minimize symptoms. And, with some education around hormones and their options, she can make requests of her doctors about her healthcare and push back if they are dismissed.

That is our mission. To give women the information and tools to empower themselves to get the help they need.

It is sad that, at a time when we are struggling, we must become warrioresses and fight hard to feel better, but the fight will be worth it if we can get better support for ourselves and lay the groundwork so that future generations of women are able to not fall into the "stress trap" that our generation is now trying to get out of. We are seeing the result of a grand-scale social experiment where women systemically took on too much stress, and the results show we haven't fared well. Let's look at how to break the cycle.

— CHAPTER 3 —

What is the Triangle of Hormonal Health?

We'd like to tell you the story of how it all began.

In 2015, Claire was on sabbatical in Australia, doing some soul searching after a challenging year. She was directionless with her work, her health was horrendous (despite doing everything she believed she should be doing based on her training), huge cracks had appeared in her marriage, and she needed a break.

During her trip, she had gone to Byron Bay with a friend.

Her friend was in the early stages of perimenopause and was recently single and had been thrown into juggling solo parenting two young children, a demanding full-time job, and trying to figure out the finances to live in one of the most expensive cities in the world. She was exhausted, overwhelmed, and at her wits' end. Her focus was not on feeding herself carefully and, understandably, she was looking for comfort in food because her reality was challenging at that moment in time. She had been experiencing debilitatingly heavy periods, and the doctor had made some suggestions that felt like a sticking-plaster approach.

As they sat on the beach chatting about this situation, Claire was trying to explain how the food, stress, and period issues were connected. In a moment of clarity, she grabbed her journal and drew a triangle to illustrate simply to her friend how the hormones being produced by her stress were exacerbated by her food and the knock-on effect that was happening with her periods. It was a lightbulb moment – for Claire as much as for her friend.

She came back from that trip and told Laura, who then dived deeply into pages and pages of research, and found that not only was this theory correct, but it was also unique. She also developed the idea that other systems such as the digestion and immune system were victims to this interplay. And thus, the Triangle of Hormonal Health was born. Little did we know that this seemingly simple explanation would lead to thousands of hours of research and tomes of documents, resulting in an international college providing training based on the model, hundreds of practitioners training in the work, thousands of clients being helped, invitations to speak on podcasts and talk at conferences, and, of course, this book!

On initial viewing, the concept might seem simple but as you dive into it, you start to see how in-depth it really is.

The reason it is brilliant (if we do say so ourselves) is that when people understand how their diet and lifestyle choices are affecting their health and when they are educated on how to make changes, they are empowered to choose differently.

We aren't naïve enough to believe that this is the root cause of every human condition, but we haven't seen someone with symptoms who has all the foundations of health in place. Often, it's not for the lack of trying on their part. We've worked with plenty of women who are up to their eyes in research and are trying everything. That was us, and the problem is that the health industry is full of conflicting information that seems to change month on month. By cutting through the white noise and fake news, and bringing the focus back to what is going on in the body hormonally, we are quickly able to see where things we've tried have failed and what to do moving forward to be in the best health we can be.

How does it work?

The human body has over 50 hormones. Some are well known and some are more obscure, but they all have an important job to do.

The medical model tends to be very segmented in its approach when looking at the body. There is no space for joined-up thinking, and the focus on treating the symptom where the symptom manifests means that the root cause is often overlooked, allowing other symptoms to spring up. The complementary therapy world is often guilty of this, too. We are aware of plenty of therapies where the therapist focuses on where the issue is manifesting but doesn't dive deeper to find out where it is truly coming from. However, the body doesn't work like this; everything works together. If one area is struggling, it puts more pressure on other areas. We are both trained kinesiology practitioners and tutors, and want to use the example of muscles as a basic example of how this concept works. If a muscle is injured and can't work properly, it puts a lot of pressure on the other muscles around it to ensure it can still perform the movement it is involved in. The same is true of hormones. A hormone that is in demand will put pressure on the other hormones and organs to ensure it can deliver and keep the body functioning.

What we need to remember is that the human body is an incredible machine. This machine has thousands of jobs but with one objective. That objective is homeostasis – the process of keeping all our complex systems in a stable condition. It will do everything possible to keep the ship steady. That is an astonishing feat. But if we aren't giving it what it needs to do that, it must work hard to maintain homeostasis, and over time this takes its toll and that is how we end up with symptoms of ill health. To be clear, we are talking about chronic conditions here, things that have built up over time because of pressure being put on our body in one way or another.

Imagine you have stubbed and broken your toe. Once the searing pain has worn off, you are likely to need to avoid putting any weight on it, so you are hobbling around, not using your toe, which means that your foot may be held at a strange angle and your other toes are doing work they don't usually do. If this goes on, over time there will be extra pressure put on your ankle, then your knee, and eventually your hip. In kinesiology, we call this a "compensation". Other systems are compensating for the muscles that can't do their job.

It's not a hip problem that you have; it's a toe problem. But your brain and body know which bit to protect, and which parts can work harder to ensure you can carry on living your life doing what living things are supposed to do – which, you might remember from Biology GCSE, is breathe, respond, reproduce, grow, eat, excrete, and move. But when there is a part of us that can't work effectively, it takes a lot of work from other parts to make sure we can function.

Hormones work in the same way that your toe, ankle, leg, and hip were working in the example. If one set of hormones can't work effectively because of a transition such as menopause or because of something we have been doing which stops them from being able to work effectively, other sets of hormones will get involved, but over time this causes more problems than are being solved.

This compensation takes up a huge amount of effort, or, as we introduced in the beginning of this book, bandwidth. And just like your internet connection, if you are taking up too much bandwidth, you have a system failure.

So, what is it?

The purpose of the Triangle of Hormonal Health is to take all the guesswork out of knowing where to start and bring you back to three vital body systems which most of us are making work far too hard, using up so much bandwidth that our body can't thrive. These systems are also where you can effect change because we have absolute control over the decisions we make in our diet and lifestyles. It's an empowering position to be in – understanding where you can make changes that will benefit your health.

The three sets of hormones it focuses on are:

- blood sugar hormones
- stress hormones
- sex hormones (our reproductive hormones).

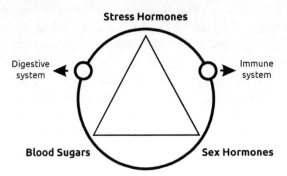

DIAGRAM I – THE TRIANGLE OF HORMONAL HEALTH

We are going to spend the first part of this book deep-diving into each of these areas so you can truly understand the impact of these hormones on your health. For now, though, let's just look at the concept.

Imagine a three-legged stool. If we want our stool to be sturdy and weight bearing, we need all three legs to be strong and stable. If one of our legs is wonky, we have an unstable stool; the other two legs can compensate, and we can prop it up, but if two or more legs are wonky, it's likely to fall over. This is a bit like our body.

If we have an issue in one set of hormones – let's say we are undergoing some major stress – we may have some low-level symptoms like headaches or insomnia that we can mostly ignore or medicate. The rest of our body can compensate for this stress and the impact it is having, and we can carry on. However, if we add eating sporadically and making poor food choices to that imbalance, we are putting pressure on another hormone system. Now, on top of those headaches, we've added unstable blood sugars, so we are likely to experience mood swings, insomnia, fatigue (the list is endless).

Of course, all those symptoms can feel unrelated, and we usually normalize them as part of life, but they are warning signs that your stool is unstable.

This is all before we start dealing with menopause, when our sex hormones are naturally going to be causing a "wonky leg" as they are fluctuating. It's now more than ever that we need our other two legs to be stable.

Relating this back to the Triangle of Hormonal Health, the stool is the triangle. Each leg is a point on the triangle and each point refers to a set of hormones – one point for blood sugars, one for stress hormones, one for our sex hormones.

These hormones interact in astonishing ways. Seemingly unrelated hormones affect body systems that you wouldn't imagine they interact with. When we start to show you how your blood sugar hormones are inextricably linked with digestion, anxiety, and stress, you will see why this model is so useful as a guide to work out where to start with your health.

You will notice that there are two arrows that point away from the triangle to the digestive system and the immune system. The reason for this is that many, many women have symptoms or conditions of the immune and digestive systems, but these are victims of the wonky stool. It's a sign that there are unstable hormones, and the knock-on effect is the development of symptoms, conditions, and ill health.

Medical issues can be really complicated. They can also be simple and unnecessarily overcomplicated, and many things can be overlooked because they can't be tested for or don't fit into the medical system of diagnosis.

Ongoing inflammation is recognized as a major cause of chronic health issues, but the medical model doesn't prioritize finding out where and why the inflammation is there; it is more important to eliminate the inflammation and stop the symptom. It's not rocket science. Your body is creating inflammation in response to something that is happening in your body; the Triangle of Hormonal Health helps to explain where that issue can be coming from.

The human body is quite basic in its needs. It needs the right fuel, water, movement, sleep, and rest. Most of the time we don't give it what it needs, and then we become frustrated when it can't function.

The triangle is a tool to show you what your body needs to create the *foundations* of health.

Not everything can be fixed, but many issues can be managed. This is not a one-size-fits-all approach, but an empowerment and management tool. It's a guide to creating real change and educating ourselves so we see our body isn't doing crazy things; it's just trying to show us what we need to change, and we can listen to it and respond. We've worked in clinic with some incredibly unwell people who have worked with the most expensive doctors, nutritionists, and therapists, and we've yet to see someone who was still experiencing symptoms when they had these foundations in place.

The best part of this process is that we can effect change in these hormone systems because they are deeply linked to lifestyle choices and diet. Menopause is going to happen regardless of our diet and lifestyle, but if we want to sail through the process, we need to stabilize our stool, and that takes understanding what to do.

You might be thinking, "My blood sugars and hormones are fine. I've had the lab tests." What we will show you in the following chapters is how overlooked and misunderstood these hormone systems are and how laboratory tests don't always give you the full picture.

— CHAPTER 4 —

Blood sugar hormones

Why blood sugars?

The most common response we hear when we talk to people about this topic is "Why wasn't I taught this before?"

This is truly our favourite thing to talk about because it is full of "aha" moments, and understanding this information is incredibly empowering.

Blood sugars are the level of glucose (sugar) present in our blood and the process by which this is maintained. This is at the core of our work because looking after our blood sugars is one of the most important things we can do to keep our body well. It doesn't sound very interesting when described in this way, but when we dive into this subject and you see the myriad of connections both with our health in general and, more specifically, during menopause, you will understand why we are passionate about spreading the word.

Due to the obesity and diabetes epidemic, most people understand what blood sugars are, and yet despite the mainstream narrative, correct blood sugar metabolism is one of the most overlooked and misunderstood processes in the human body, However, stable blood sugar hormones are fundamental to our health.

Let's come back to bandwidth. We don't have enough bandwidth during perimenopause, so we need to look at ways to free some up. The biggest stressors that take up our bandwidth are those we must deal with repeatedly. Obvious examples would be smoking, alcoholism, or drug addictions. However, the standard Western diet and today's busy lifestyle are also major stressors on the body because they destabilize blood sugars.

We love talking about blood sugars because, with a little bit of education, we can make dietary changes that have a huge impact on our health, and these benefits can be felt quickly. By reducing blood sugar imbalances, we are literally freeing up bandwidth in the body, which creates more resilience. In turn, it is possible to reduce minor symptoms that are muddying our health "picture" and we can focus on the deeper issues caused by our menopause. More advanced symptoms such as insulin resistance, prediabetes and type 2 diabetes may take longer to resolve, but they have been shown to be reversible with correct diet and lifestyle choices.

While many people are aware that diet and food choices play a role in maintaining optimum blood sugars, many people are unaware that other factors such as lifestyle, poor protein sources, and food intolerance also determine whether blood sugars remain stable.

One of the reasons blood sugar instabilities are so misunderstood is because of the way they are tested by the medical model.

The standard medical tests for blood sugar instabilities are glucose tests (finger prick tests), fasting glucose tests (blood test), glucose tolerance testing, and urine testing.

- Finger prick tests will show the level of sugar in your blood at the moment the test is taken.

- Fasting blood sugar tests will show how your body is coping under the stress of fasting.

- Glucose tolerance tests will show if your body is responding appropriately to sugar.

- Urine testing shows if the kidneys are becoming damaged due to high blood sugar levels.

- HbA1C tests show how "sugary" your blood has become.

All these tests measure blood sugar levels and responses. None of them measures insulin, the hormone that manages blood sugar levels, and its effectiveness at doing its job.

This is very important when we come back to the body's priority being homeostasis and keeping the internal state of the body steady by any means possible. For blood sugar stabilization, there are two primary hormones: insulin and glucagon, which are both produced by the pancreas.

The pancreas has two major functions. It has an endocrine function (translated as "it secretes hormones") and it has a digestive function. It produces enzymes that help us digest our food and break the fats down so that fat-soluble vitamins like vitamin D can be absorbed. Interestingly, 95 per cent of its function is dedicated to digestion and only 5 per cent is supposed to be involved with blood sugar balancing.

When we have unstable blood sugars, the pancreas is constantly put into action to deal with this crisis instead of doing its digestive job, and over time this is unsustainable.

These tests therefore aren't showing how well your blood sugars function, how hard they are working and how much bandwidth is being taken up to maintain the correct blood sugar balance. If the pancreas is having to work hard, it is a major cause of underlying stress in our body, and this stress contributes to a myriad of physical and emotional symptoms.

The other issue is that many people (including the medical model) assume that just because we have eaten something, our blood sugars will be regulated. This couldn't be further from the truth. The example of diabetics who experience low blood sugar being told to eat something sweet shows a massive misunderstanding of how to create blood sugar stabilization and future resilience. This short-sighted correction can lead to further problems later in the day. What is needed is an understanding of what to eat and when to eat to avoid the lows (or highs) in the first place.

Many people choose to wear a continuous glucose monitor to check what is happening with blood sugars, and this data is very useful but, again, it doesn't show how hard the body is working to keep the blood sugars stable.

During perimenopause and post-menopause, blood sugar balancing becomes essential if we want to manage symptoms effectively, regardless of whether we are using HRT.

Insulin resistance is a commonplace health issue driven by our modern lifestyles. Thanks to our high-carbohydrate, ultra-processed diets, our poor pancreases are constantly being required to make more and more insulin. Eventually, the organ gives up and the body's cells no longer respond properly to the insulin that the body makes. Insulin resistance is one of the pillars of metabolic dysfunction, alongside obesity (especially around the middle), high cholesterol, high triglycerides, fatty liver, and high blood pressure. A staggering 33 per cent of the population now have metabolic disorder.

But the blood tests also don't show what is happening with insulin, so the picture we receive from testing is skewed and we have normalized these issues.

What is fascinating is that insulin resistance naturally occurs in puberty, pregnancy, and perimenopause and is, in fact, beneficial in puberty and pregnancy to allow growth to happen at these important stages of life. But it is not beneficial in perimenopause or menopause when both high and low oestrogen, depending on the stage of the process you are in, will contribute to insulin resistance. If we can balance our blood sugars, we can support the pancreas, insulin production, and the menopausal process.

Menopause as a hormonal transition doesn't happen in isolation. It affects other hormone systems, which is why we can experience such far-reaching and seemingly unrelated symptoms. Behind many of these symptoms is insulin resistance and unstable blood sugars.

To get a deeper understanding of what is happening, we need to dive into the science bit and get nerdy about blood sugar hormones...

What are the blood sugar hormones and how do they work?

One of the big "aha" moments we had in our journey and that we enjoy sharing with others is this realization:

Every time we put food into our mouths, we have a hormonal reaction.

It's an important concept. Because when we understand it, we see food in a whole new light, and it blows apart the doctrine of "calories in, calories out". It explains why many women fail to lose weight using modern diets, and later in the book we are going to talk about what to do instead.

Because it's so important and to make sure it lands, we are going to say it again:

Every time we put food into our mouths, we have a hormonal reaction.

And that reaction can take us either towards wellness or towards poor health. Which way we head depends on which hormones are produced when we eat. It is therefore useful to understand these hormones because many symptoms experienced by menopausal women can be attributed to imbalances here.

There are eight hormones that work together with regard to blood sugar and diet:

- glucagon
- insulin
- ghrelin
- cholecystokinin (CCK)
- leptin
- somatostatin
- amylin
- cortisol.

Glucagon and insulin

These hormones do opposite jobs but work together. When our blood sugars rise, the pancreas produces insulin to lower the blood sugar by telling the body to absorb the glucose and store it in our liver, muscles, and fat cells.

When our blood sugars fall, our pancreas produces glucagon, a hormone which tells the liver to send the glucose back into the blood because energy is required.

This hormone interplay is useful to understand because it shows the relationship between what we eat and fat storage. One of the important roles of insulin is to signal the body to store fat. In fact, a fat cell *cannot* grow in the absence of insulin.

This is a clever survival strategy of the body. In our primal ancestry, when we were cavemen, carbohydrates and sugars would have been scarce, so the body would store energy in fat cells to be used in the event of an energy shortage.

Low insulin will make us feel fatigued and anxious. High insulin triggers the body to produce oestrogen but reduces libido.

We are going to be exploring a lot more about insulin during this chapter because high insulin is behind many chronic issues that humans are struggling with today.

Ghrelin

Ghrelin is our hunger hormone produced by cells in the gut, especially the stomach. Blood levels of ghrelin are highest before meals when we are hungry, and when it is at its highest, we experience hunger pangs and tummy rumbling. After we eat, ghrelin stops being released, and levels drop. They slowly rise over the next three hours; once they have built up, we experience the hunger signals again. Ghrelin is connected to anxiety because of its correlation to hunger. If our body perceives we are hungry because we haven't eaten enough nutrient-dense foods, we will experience anxiety.

There is a connection between ghrelin and inflammation as ghrelin increases the production of cells that suppress and calm the immune system. This is one of the explanations of why fasting has been shown to be a supportive method for conditions such as autoimmunity, which is an overly stimulated immune system.

Balanced ghrelin stimulates libido.

Cholecystokinin (CCK)

Cholecystokinin (commonly known as CCK) is our satisfaction and appetite hormone secreted by cells in the small intestine. It stimulates the release of bile from the gallbladder into the small intestine to digest our fats. It also signals to the pancreas to secrete enzymes for digestion, as well as slowing the transit of broken-down food (chyme) through the small intestine so we can absorb the nutrients. When we don't have the right amount of CCK, we will experience issues with gut motility, IBS, and bloating!

CCK also plays a role in behaviour regulation and sexual behaviour, and there is evidence that if CCK is imbalanced, it can contribute to increased anxiety, panic, and poor memory.

CCK is reduced in people with obesity.

Leptin

Leptin is a hormone produced in the fat cells in the small intestine that inhibits hunger and promotes fat burning.

Leptin turns glycogen (stored glucose) back into glucose, which in turn fuels our cells and muscles and gives us more energy. It's a hunger inhibiter so reduces appetite and cravings.

Leptin is super sensitive to starchy carbohydrates. More starchy carbs equal more leptin. The level of leptin in our blood is also directly related to how much body fat we have. In other words, the more fat you have, the more leptin you have. However, in obesity, where someone would have high levels of leptin and should have a reduced appetite and cravings, we see a condition called *leptin resistance*. This is a situation where there are high levels of leptin, but the body is not responding to it, so hunger is elevated and fat burn is inhibited. With leptin resistance, we also have reduced libido, poor sleep, and susceptibility to infections.

Leptin also has a role in the immune system. High levels of leptin can increase inflammation which can contribute to cholesterol issues, IBS, heart disease, autoimmune conditions, skin issues, and cancer. If leptin is high, we also experience more pain.

Somatostatin

The primary function of somatostatin is to prevent the production of other hormones in the endocrine and exocrine system. Somatostatin turns off the flow of certain hormones and secretions when your body doesn't need them any more.

With regard to blood sugars, somatostatin is like our stop valve: it keeps everything in check to maintain homeostasis. It responds well to fat in the diet.

Low levels of somatostatin have been linked to conditions such as Alzheimer's.

Amylin

Amylin helps control blood glucose levels along with insulin. Amylin and insulin are partners, and when amylin is working properly, the body needs less insulin. Amylin signals the stomach to slow food movement into the small intestine (gastric/stomach emptying), which helps with the feeling of being full and satiated. Amylin plays a role in healthy weight maintenance because of this fullness effect, as well as increasing leptin sensitivity which stimulates fat burning and inhibits hunger.

Cortisol

Cortisol is not technically a blood sugar hormone; it is a stress hormone. But it has a massive effect on our blood sugar hormones. One of its jobs is to flood the body with glucose to prepare it for the fight-or-flight response. Simply put, it releases sugar into our bloodstream and muscles so we can run away from danger. But the problem is that while the perceived danger can be because something dangerous is happening, more commonly it is because of the following:

- We are experiencing general stress in our day.
- Our blood sugar has dropped too low, either because we are hungry or because it has crashed after we produced a load of insulin to deal with the muffin we had with our morning coffee.
- We have eaten something we are intolerant to, which is now causing us to have an adrenaline and cortisol reaction.

To understand why this is happening let's look at the blood sugar rollercoaster.

Blood sugar metabolism and the blood sugar rollercoaster

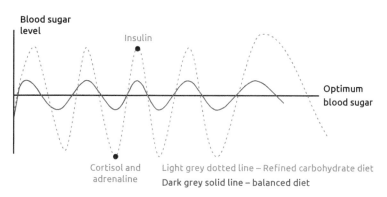

DIAGRAM 2 – THE BLOOD SUGAR ROLLERCOASTER

Let's bring blood sugar hormones to life! As you have learned from previous pages, when we eat, our blood sugars rise, and insulin brings them back down again. What we eat determines how high they rise.

Blood sugar goes up, insulin is secreted, glucose becomes glycogen, and blood sugar goes down.

Normal blood sugar metabolism

Blood sugar ↑, we secrete insulin = blood sugar ↓ and convert glucose to glycogen

> Blood sugars ↓, we secrete adrenaline + glucagon which converts glyco-gen to glucose = blood sugar ↑

If you look at the diagram above, you will see the nice gentle wave that represents optimum blood sugar. Many people are not metabolizing their food in this way, however, and instead are experiencing the peaks and troughs of the blood sugar rollercoaster.

When we eat something high in carbohydrates, the glucose saturates our cells and sends our blood sugar levels soaring, which triggers insulin to be secreted, which then causes blood sugars to crash.

The body often produces excessive insulin in preparation for the next large requirement of insulin, bringing down our blood sugar level, often below normal range. This drop in blood sugars is stressful and triggers a release of our flight-or-fight responses, adrenaline and cortisol. This release creates carb cravings and forces us to go and forage for sugar, which drives our blood sugars back up again, often higher than is optimal. This in turn leads us to create more insulin, and the cycle continues.

Constant insulin production causes the mechanism for fat burning to switch off and fat storage to switch on, which can lead to significant amounts of weight gain.

This blood sugar rollercoaster can also lead to heightened anxiety, a loss of higher brain function, and increased hunger. So it doesn't matter how much willpower you think you have, if your hormones are signalling you must have sugar and you must have it now, you are going to go and eat that cake.

What do we mean by a diet that is high in carbohydrates?

Most people know that junk food and processed foods are high in sugar and trans fats. What is often misunderstood is that a "normal, healthy" diet can be equally high in carbohydrates.

An example of this would be:

- Breakfast is a bowl of muesli, a glass of orange juice and a fruit yogurt.

- Lunch is a salad with a sweet potato.

- Fruit for an afternoon snack.

- Dinner is a fish risotto with butternut squash and some dark chocolate.

All good healthy, natural food. But this is a carbohydrate-heavy diet, and this will be contributing to a blood sugar rollercoaster effect. It doesn't matter what the source of the carbohydrate is, whether it's a carrot or carrot cake. Once it is broken down and hits the bloodstream, it becomes glucose.

Too much of this rollercoaster and we end up with too much insulin in our system.

Hyperinsulinism

In the modern age, with an abundance of carbohydrates at our fingertips, we are now seeing insulin signalling for fat storage as a growing problem as it is contributing to issues such as diabetes and obesity.

When there is a consistently high level of sugar in the diet, it requires frequent insulin production. Every cell in our body has a receptor cell for insulin. When the body is constantly flooded with insulin, these receptor cells become insensitive to insulin. This is called *insulin resistance*. Insulin is no longer doing the job of lowering blood sugar. This creates a condition called *hyperinsulinism*, which is the precursor to type 2 diabetes.

Hyperinsulinism blood sugar metabolism

Hyperinsulinism = Blood sugar ↑ and insulin ↑

The body is now trying to deal with the huge amount of unused, unabsorbed insulin, and we start to crave carbohydrates.

In menopause, as reproductive hormone levels fluctuate, the body can become less responsive to insulin, and hyperinsulinism can be common – hence the connection with menopause, weight gain, and blood sugar instability.

Obesity and diabetes are caused by insulin resistance. The medical profession agree that insulin resistance is driven by three factors: inflammation, stress, and hyperinsulinism (too much insulin caused by poor diet choices).

Doctors use medication to reduce inflammation and blood sugars, but information emerging from the leaders in metabolic science, such as Dr Ben Bikman, is now proving that the medications really don't work and are even contributing to making the situation worse because they are toxic at a cellular level. Because of this, more and more progressive medical practitioners have realized that the only feasible route to dealing with the epidemic of blood sugar issues is diet. However, none of them are targeting inflammation and stress, which, medically, are considered too intangible to tackle head on or require coaching about lifestyle choices; these are no longer the realm of the GP and therefore are not areas that are really explored.

What is diabetes?

Diabetes becomes a common issue with menopause as the hormonal changes that start in perimenopause can disrupt blood sugar levels and put some women at higher risk of type 2 diabetes or make diabetes harder to manage. But there can often be some confusion about diabetes.

There are two types of diabetes:

- Type 1 = irreversible pancreatic damage either from a defect at birth or brought on by an autoimmune response. The pancreas is unable to make insulin because the islets of Langerhans, where insulin is made, are either missing or no longer functional.

- Type 2 = a condition brought about when the body has spent too long in hyperinsulinism due to a high-stress lifestyle and/or a high-carbohydrate diet where the pancreas can no longer produce insulin.

Diabetes blood sugar metabolism

Diabetes = Blood sugar ↑ = insulin ↓

Once we are in this place, we are unable to process any sugar out of the body without medication or insulin replacement. There are multiple life-limiting side effects that accompany diabetes, and it is a challenging condition to deal with.

However, there is a lot of research that shows that type 2 diabetes can be reversed with the right diet, changing some aspects of lifestyle, and finding the right exercise.

Another important aspect to consider with the blood sugar rollercoaster is skipping meals. Skipping meals can cause our blood sugars to drop too low, creating a sense of anxiety. Only by eating in a balanced way and regularly can we relieve the body of this stress cycle.

Many people extol the virtues of fasting. The science is pretty resolute that it is good for us, but if we have unstable blood sugars, we are creating more stress in the body, so we need to focus on balancing blood sugars for a few months first before doing any fasting.

One of the fascinating aspects of blood sugar hormones is how they interact with other systems such as the digestion and the immune system. When our blood sugar hormones are imbalanced, we often see issues in these other areas.

Most people will know the common conditions connected with blood sugar imbalances such as obesity and diabetes, and often we connect other symptoms such as feeling "hangry" or shaky if our blood sugars drop too low. However, many of the major symptoms associated with blood sugar hormone imbalances are totally overlooked and, worse, often diagnosed as other conditions. Some of these diagnoses can result in the prescription of unnecessary medications that have big side effects. In these instances, it is common to hear that the medical practitioners making the diagnosis and offering the prescription have never looked at diet or queried underlying blood sugar imbalances.

But insulin resistance, obesity, and diabetes are not the only issues associated with blood sugars imbalances. There are now a variety of conditions associated with blood sugar imbalances. Many, many thought leaders in the medical and biochemical realms agree that dementia, Alzheimer's disease, PCOS, migraines, erectile dysfunction, skin tags, fatty liver, certain cancers, gout, arthritis, osteoarthritis, heart disease, high blood pressure, and sarcopenia have their roots in blood sugar imbalances caused by stress, ultra-processed food, seed oils, increased carbohydrates and low-protein diets, and being sedentary. In fact, dementia is commonly referred to as "diabetes type 3".

This is an incredibly sobering list.

We can break it down further to look at which hormones are behind common issues.

Symptoms associated with blood sugar hormones

Linked to leptin imbalance	Linked to insulin imbalance	Linked to cholecystokinin imbalance	Linked to ghrelin imbalance
Increased appetite	High blood pressure and rapid heartbeat	Upper abdominal pain	Increased appetite
Obesity	Low HDL cholesterol	Nausea	Eating disorders such as anorexia
Belly fat	Skin tags	Light-headedness	Lack of appetite
Fatigue	Increased waistline	Heartburn	IBS
Pain disorders such as fibromyalgia and joint pain	High triglycerides	Gut motility issues	Gastrointestinal conditions such as gastritis, irritable bowel syndrome, celiac, inflammatory bowel disease
	Blurred vision	Anxiety	
Cravings	Headaches and migraines	Digestive issues such as bloating, constipation, and irritable bowel syndrome	
Increased inflammation	Frequent infections and immune issues including allergies and food intolerances		Heart disease
Poor fertility	Brain fog and difficulty concentrating	Gallbladder issues	Muscle atrophy
Mood disorders including depression and anxiety	Fatigue	Increased appetite	Weak bones
	PCOS and hormone imbalance	Difficulty losing weight	Pancreatitis
	Mood disorders including depression and anxiety		Increased inflammation
	Behavioural issues		Low stomach acid
	Insomnia – either trouble falling asleep or waking in the night		Anxiety
	Diabetes		Poor fertility
			Increased stress

Constant snacking and grazing is a symptom caused in part by the "protein leverage hypothesis".[1] This fascinating work explores how mammals will keep eating until they have had enough protein.

Although this hasn't yet been proven, it is an interesting lens through which to view this list of symptoms. For example, a feeling of deep hunger or lack of food can result in anxiety. If we have covered the obvious feeling by overeating carbs but are protein deficient, that anxiety could still have far-reaching effects.

Common symptoms associated with menopause that are exacerbated by blood sugar imbalances include:

- allergies
- anxiety
- bloating
- blood pressure imbalances
- brain fog (menofog)
- depression
- dizziness
- electric shock sensation
- fatigue
- fluid retention
- high cholesterol
- high triglycerides
- incontinence
- insomnia
- irregular heartbeat
- itchy skin
- joint pain
- loss of libido
- mood swings
- night sweats
- panic disorder
- poor memory
- tingling extremities
- urinary tract infection
- weight gain.

Menopausal women are commonly prescribed medications such as antidepressants and anti-anxiety medications, as well as medications for heartburn, constipation, insomnia, migraines, joint pain, heartbeat irregularities, blood pressure irregularities, cholesterol, blood sugars, and triglycerides.

In some cases, these issues even lead to invasive surgery. We are not saying that changing your diet will miraculously make these issues go away, but most people report a change in the severity of symptoms, and if you're faced with the option of potentially dangerous medication or surgery, you've got nothing to lose by tweaking your diet to see if that helps first.

What causes blood sugar instability?

Blood sugar hormones are meant to fluctuate throughout the day. However, blood sugar instability is one of the underlying causes of hormonal symptoms, and it is one of the first places we focus on to improve the wellbeing of a menopausal woman.

Carbohydrate excess

As we have stated, eating a diet high in carbohydrates and skipping meals are common causes of blood sugar instability.

What is a high-carbohydrate food? We can use the Harvard University's "table of glycaemic load"[2] which shows how much sugar is deposited in the body after eating a specific food. Sugar (sucrose) is the benchmark and rates at 100 out of 100, but some surprising foods come in high on the scale, many of which are often considered healthy options:

- cornflakes 93/100
- white rice 89/100
- rice cakes 82/100

- white baguette 95/100
- baked potato 111/100
- mashed potato 87/100.

While eating too many carbohydrates is an issue, eating carbohydrates on their own is also a major problem.

Imagine a helium balloon. If that helium balloon isn't weighted down and we let go of it, it's going to fly up in the air. That's what carbohydrates do to our blood sugars: they send them soaring, and we need to "weight them down". We do that by eating our carbohydrates in the right ratio with proteins and fats.

However, carbohydrates and skipping meals aren't the only cause of blood sugars spiking. There are some other culprits.

Eating low-fat diets

Fat is an essential macronutrient that is needed to produce cholesterol, which is used to make our reproductive hormones. Fat also stabilizes blood sugars as it slows down our digestion. Low-fat diet alternative foods are often high in carbohydrates, which imbalances blood sugars.

Protein deficiency

Protein helps stabilize blood sugars by blunting the absorption of carbohydrates. As protein breaks down into glucose more slowly than carbohydrate, the effect of protein on blood glucose levels tends to be over a longer time. Many modern diets are low in quality protein.

Micronutrient deficiency

There are important micronutrients (such as vitamins and minerals) that are needed for blood sugar metabolism. These include zinc and magnesium, which act like the doorkeeper to the cell allowing glucose to enter and exit. If we have a diet low in these nutrients, we could have blood sugar instability.

Stress

Stressful situations require our bodies to produce stress hormones including cortisol, which has a knock-on effect on blood sugar levels. When stressed, the body prepares itself by ensuring that enough sugar or energy is readily available to deal with the situation.

When our blood sugar hormones drop, adrenaline and cortisol rise, creating more stress in the body.

Infection and illness

Infection is stressful for the body. When your body is fighting an illness, your organs require more energy to battle the invading pathogen. So as part of the body's natural defence mechanism, more glucose is released into the bloodstream.

Activity and exercise

Our blood sugar hormones are connected to exercise because we need glucose for energy to be able to move our bodies. When we work out, insulin goes down, so more glucose is released from the liver for fuel.

However, insulin can also increase in response to stress hormones produced during more strenuous types of exercise such as weightlifting, sprints, and competitive sports, so blood sugar stability is dependent on the style of exercise we do and the amount we do it. Cortisol is naturally higher earlier in the day, falls throughout the day, and is lowest at night. If we are doing workout classes later in the evening and producing cortisol, this could create an insulin spike and imbalance blood sugar hormones.

Food intolerances

Food allergies and intolerances create inflammation in the gut, which is stressful for the body and produces adrenaline/cortisol in response. If you eat food you are intolerant to, you may feel your heart start to race, for example. This is a stress response caused by your food choice.

Poor gut environment

Poor gut health increases the risk of insulin resistance. It is stressful for the body to have an impaired digestive function, and this creates a cortisol response. If the gut tissue becomes inflamed and damaged with particles of food, known as endotoxins, entering the bloodstream, this triggers the immune system into thinking a foreign body is in the bloodstream and creates inflammation – cortisol and a release of insulin. More on the gut later.

Menopause

The relationship between insulin and the reproductive hormones, oestrogen, progesterone, and testosterone, is a back-and-forth dynamic.

Increased insulin leads to increased adrenaline and cortisol levels, which will cause the body to deplete progesterone. Increased insulin also leads to increased oestrogen production.

On the flip side, oestrogen and progesterone influence the way insulin works in the body – for example, oestrogen helps to optimize insulin.

Typically, perimenopausal women who have higher levels of oestrogen have increased insulin sensitivity, and post-menopausal women who have reduced oestrogen levels have increased insulin resistance.

This interplay is at the core of the Triangle of Hormonal Health we discussed earlier. Remember the wonky stool?

Dehydration

Your blood needs adequate levels of water in it to maintain an ideal ratio of water to glucose, and therefore dehydration can easily spike blood sugar hormones if glucose is concentrated. Drinking water also helps your kidneys flush out excess sugar.

Medications including the birth control pill

The high levels of hormones in the pill cause spikes in insulin levels. On top of this, not having a natural cycle is stressful for the body, therefore producing cortisol and spikes in blood sugar hormones.

Other medications that affect blood sugar stability include oral corticosteroids and statins, which increase blood sugar levels by:

- causing the liver to release more glucose

- stopping glucose being absorbed from the blood by the muscle and fat cells

- reducing the body's sensitivity to insulin.

Lack of sleep

Like so many functions in the body, sleep and blood sugars are entwined with each other. Sleep affects blood sugar hormones, and blood sugar hormones affect our sleep.

Sleep deprivation is incredibly stressful and inflammatory for the body, causing an increase in both cortisol and insulin production. In turn, if you are eating a carbohydrate-heavy diet, the sugar in your blood will fall at night, which triggers cortisol, and this will wake you up.

Stimulants and recreational drugs

Stimulants such as coffee, tea, alcohol, and smoking all raise blood pressure, create cortisol and adrenaline, and in turn raise insulin. Any foods, drinks, or substances that give us an adrenaline kick will be creating a blood sugar rollercoaster. And the difficulty is that the more we consume these substances, the more we crave and rely on them when our blood sugars fall.

> **TAKE-HOME MESSAGE**
> Blood sugars are one of the most fundamentally important aspects of human health. It is imperative that we keep them balanced, and given how many factors can affect them, we often must work harder to keep them balanced so that we have solid foundations for our health. With blood sugars having such a huge impact on our hormonal health, how can we expect HRT to be the magic bullet that makes all our menopausal symptoms disappear?

How many of these factors are influencing your blood sugars? We recommend creating your own list of causes of blood sugar instability. In Part Two, we will be detailing all the ways you can address blood sugar instability including diet, nutrition supplementation, and lifestyle factors.

The Triangle of Hormonal Health and how it is affected by blood sugars

Blood sugars are the absolute foundation of the triangle. There are three main reasons for this:

First, diet is the easiest, cheapest, and quickest part of our lifestyle to change.

Second, blood sugar hormones are connected to many other systems and hormones.

Third, having stable blood sugars and blood sugar hormones is an absolute foundation for good health. So many other symptoms will change when this part of the puzzle is in place. And the benefits of getting this sorted are manifold. It makes it easier as a clinician to get a real idea of what is going on when it's not clouded by symptoms caused by unstable blood sugars. We can literally see the wood for the trees. Women feel better and more energized and are encouraged to continue the path. They are saving money on unnecessary supplements and faddy foodstuffs, and they feel educated and empowered. It's a real win-win.

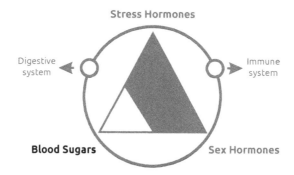

DIAGRAM 3 – BLOOD SUGARS AND THE TRIANGLE OF HORMONAL HEALTH

During menopause, our sex hormones "leg" is going to be wonky by nature and, with the pressures of life and work, we may not be able to change much about our stress, but with blood sugars, we can make change immediately.

If our blood sugars are unstable, we are wasting money on fancy supplements and our HRT may be ineffective – in fact, while everything we do towards our "wellness" is great, most of it will be a sticking plaster. We need to create deep foundations if we want to build a house. Stabilizing our blood sugars is how we create those foundations, and by shoring up that leg, we can even reduce issues in the other legs. We are going to look more deeply into what is happening with all the hormones in subsequent chapters but as an overview, if we have unstable blood sugars, we can expect the following.

Stress hormones
When we have low blood sugar, we produce adrenaline and cortisol.

Imbalanced blood sugar hormones will contribute to anxiety and mental health issues due to the activity of the actual blood sugar hormones.

Imbalanced blood sugars confuse our hunger and satisfaction levels, affecting our appetite. They also affect libido and energy.

Sex hormones
High levels of insulin in our system imbalance sex hormones, which in turn reduces our body's ability to use insulin. This contributes to weight gain and other symptoms.

Digestive function
Because of the pancreas's dual role of digestion and blood sugar management, when the pancreas is overworked from unstable blood sugars, this will cause issues in the digestive system.

Immune function
When our blood sugars are unstable, we can be susceptible to increased chronic inflammation and conditions such as autoimmune disease.

TAKE-HOME MESSAGE
Having stable blood sugars is an absolute game changer for hormones and can alleviate many common symptoms in menopause. We hope you have had some aha moments reading this chapter. An important part of this book is enabling you to join the dots between hormonal interplay, the food we eat, the lifestyle we live, and the health of our body.

Here are the key points to remember as we continue through this book:

- Blood sugar balancing can be speedy – in fact, you can improve your blood sugars with your next meal choice.

- Blood sugar hormones affect our stress hormones, sex hormones, digestive system, immune system, and our mental health.

- Insulin resistance is behind many major chronic conditions.

- All carbohydrates turn to sugar in the body.

- A baked potato deposits more sugar in the body than white sugar. Wholesome, natural foods are important, but it's just as important to monitor the carbohydrate amount you are eating.

- Menopause is not just about oestrogen or taking HRT. There are many other hormone interplays and health factors to consider.

- Eating foods we are intolerant to leads to increased cortisol and increased insulin.

See you in the next chapter where we are going to explore stress, cortisol, and the impact this can have on the menopause.

— CHAPTER 5 —

Stress hormones

Stress has become a very overused word, so much so that it now gets bandied around as a type of trophy. We have glorified being busy and somehow equate this to being successful, validated, and needed.

The impact of stress is one of the greatest threats to public health globally, and although a doctor may ask if you've been stressed, there are no key metrics to assess stress, and the effect of cumulative stress as a co-factor in chronic health conditions is rarely cited.

A UK-wide survey in 2018 revealed that 81 per cent of UK women have felt so stressed at some point that they became overwhelmed or unable to cope.[1]

What do we mean by stress? We all know the word, but it is useful to be definitive. Stress is "a state of worry or mental tension caused by a difficult situation ... a natural human response that prompts us to address challenges and threats in our lives".[2] In other words, it is our response to challenges and difficulty.

The stress response is a vital system in the body and one of the keys to our survival. In small doses, stress has many advantages. For instance, stress can help you accomplish tasks more efficiently, boost memory, improve heart function, and protect your body from infection. It is the physical stress of weight bearing that creates strength in our bones.

Some studies have shown that individuals who experienced moderate levels of stress before surgery recovered faster than individuals who had low or high levels.[3] It is true that humans have evolved to withstand some stress, but what we are dealing with today is far beyond the limit of what we can thrive in.

Historically, all the stress we experienced was acute and would include situations such as being chased by an animal or being injured navigating difficult terrain. During events such as these, the fight-or-flight response was activated, and the hormones cortisol and adrenaline worked together to ensure our survival. At the end of the event, you were either dead or alive and safe – in both cases, there was no need for the body to continue to produce stress hormones and, if alive and safe, we would enter a recovery phase.

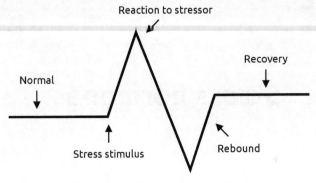

DIAGRAM 4 – THE STRESS RESPONSE PROCESS

Chronic modern stress is an unrelenting event that never ends. It can exist at a low level– for example, enduring the treadmill of work, raising children, and juggling money worries. It can be moderate, such as studying for an exam or a specific time-related concern, or it can be very high, such as a challenging divorce, moving to a new house, or a death in the family.

Moderate- and high-stress periods may come to an end, but we never truly get to the point of recovery as we are always returning to a state of low to moderate stress.

When we don't have time to recover, we are in a position of continual stress, which eventually can lead to burnout. Many women today live with this low level of burnout, and it is only with the onset of perimenopause and the changes in sex hormones that the chronic stress they have been living with for decades becomes apparent.

This continuous burnout situation has created a profound mismatch between how we are genetically designed to live and the modern experience of life. This mismatch is driving an epidemic of inflammatory diseases such as autoimmune disorders that we are seeing globally. Essentially, our highly sensitive endocrine system is not evolving fast enough to cope with the stress put upon it. The lifestyle we have created of "modern convenience" is slowly killing us.

When we talk about stress, we tend only to focus on the obvious sources of stress such as work, financial pressure, parenting, relationships, and the factors that are placed on our body just by being alive in today's environment. For this reason, instead of using the word "stress", we prefer to use the word "stressors" to make a clear distinction.

In today's world, stressors are literally everywhere. Living in the modern age is basically like swimming through a sea of stressors and hoping we survive. These stressors are taking up an extraordinary amount of our bandwidth.

Let's look at what these stressors are. The easiest way to approach this is to divide them up into the aspects of the body that they affect.

In kinesiology, we call these aspects "body realms". These essentially are different areas of the body that can be affected by different stimuli. We refer to these realms using the acronym BEES:

- B – Biochemical – stressors that are caused by chemicals we encounter in day-to-day life, and biochemical reactions in the body.

- E – Emotional – stressors caused by emotional factors.

- E – Electrical – Stressors caused by electrical stimuli or stressors affecting our body's internal electrical systems.

- S – Structural – stressors causing structural imbalances in the body or existing structural issues exacerbating stress.

Biochemical stressors

- Food intolerances
- Chemical toxicity – skin care, cleaning products, pesticides, and pollution
- Poor diet and high sugar intake
- Depleted nutrition in soils – lack of nutrients such as magnesium
- Dehydration and poor-quality water
- Medications, contraception, HRT
- Stimulants such as caffeine, alcohol, and nicotine
- Reduced sunlight and vitamin D exposure
- Radiation from nuclear fallout
- Cosmic radiation
- Chemical outgassing from furniture, carpets, etc.
- Processed food

Emotional stressors

- Anxiety
- Depression
- Overwhelm
- Relationships
- Societal pressures
- Family concerns
- Body image
- Social media pressure
- Low self-esteem
- Financial and work pressure
- Addictions

Electrical stressors

- Electromagnetic radiation including microwaves, TV, and device exposure
- Light toxicity
- Geopathic stress

Structural stressors

- Poor posture
- Lack of exercise
- Sedentary lifestyles
- Over-exercise or wrong exercise
- Restrictive clothing and shoes
- Painful conditions in muscles, organs, body systems, and joints

This picture is sobering when looked at in its entirety. It's little wonder, then, that our bodies are struggling, when, each day, we are walking through life being bombarded with these stressors.

Let's look at what happens in the body when we are stressed.

The stress response is produced by our glandular system, which is called the endocrine system. Our endocrine system is a series of glands that create hormones, our body's chemical messengers. The endocrine system works closely with our nervous system, which transmits messages through nerves electrically.

To explain this further, the endocrine system produces hormones, in response to stimulus. For example, when it's dark, a gland sends a message to begin the sleep cycle; when we really need a wee, there is a chemical message sent from our bladder to a gland in the endocrine system, which in turn makes another hormone or message to inform us we need to go to the loo; when we are hungry, a few different hormones tell the same gland we are hungry so the gland can send another chemical message to get us to go and eat something. There are thousands of these messages a day: it's light so it's time to wake up; it's dark so it's time to go to sleep; it's time to ovulate; I need to digest food; I feel safe, so I can relax; I feel scared, so I need to stay alert. All of these are chemical messages that are sent through the blood and regulated by our endocrine system. These chemical messages work slowly over time and are used to certain rhythms such as mealtimes and the shift from day to night.

Our nervous system is different. It sends messages in response to things it picks up through our senses. If we see a glass about to fall over, the nerves send messages to our hands to try to grab it. If we hear a loud bang, we react to see if we need to get out of the way of danger. Or we might smell fire or feel something that is too hot and therefore dangerous.

But our nervous system also communicates with our endocrine system if we are dealing with a lot of dangerous situations, because this will change what hormones we need.

We'd like to explain this to you in more depth so you can fully understand why stress is such a problem. To do that, we need to know the names of the glands and what they do.

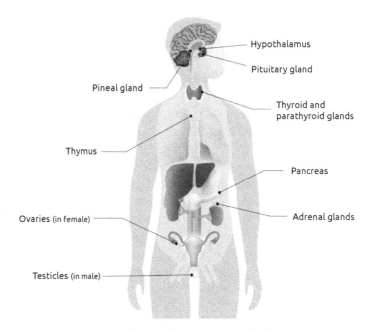

DIAGRAM 5 – THE ENDOCRINE SYSTEM

Starting at the top of the diagram and working down:

Pineal gland: This gland is affected by light and dark and regulates our sleep/wake cycle. It also has an impact on female sex hormones and the cardiovascular system. In the presence of stress, the sleep/wake cycle becomes disturbed, and we can experience sleep issues and period issues.

Hypothalamus: This isn't a gland at all but is a structure in the brain that is like your control room. It receives electrical impulses from the nervous system and communicates with other endocrine glands. In the presence of stress, the hypothalamus will be on high alert.

Pituitary gland: Known as the master gland, the pituitary is the leader of the whole endocrine orchestra. It monitors and regulates multiple functions and systems, and most of the hormonal communication comes through the pituitary gland. When the pituitary is in the presence of constant stress, we can experience memory issues and confusion.

Thyroid gland: The thyroid is in the lower front of your neck and is shaped like a butterfly. The thyroid is an important gland in the endocrine system and directly impacts the brain, digestion, metabolism, temperature, liver, gallbladder, blood sugars, bone health, and cardiovascular system. Because of the relationship between the glands in the endocrine system, the thyroid is incredibly sensitive to stress.

One in eight women will develop a thyroid disorder in their lifetime, and it is common for this to happen during the menopause transition. This can make the experience even more challenging.

An important role of the thyroid is to convert iodine into thyroid hormones triiodothyronine (T3) and thyroxine (T4). We get iodine in our diets from fish, seaweed, and dairy products, and with the nutritional depletion of our soil and the rise in popularity of veganism and dairy intolerance, it is common to have a deficiency of iodine.

T4 is the inactive form of the thyroid hormone, and it must be converted into the active form T3 before the body can use it. Some T3 is produced in your thyroid, and the body converts T4 to T3 in the liver, gut, kidneys, and brain, so keeping these organs healthy and functioning is an important part of keeping your thyroid happy.

In the presence of regular stress, thyroid function is lowered and the conversion of T4 to T3 is inhibited.

Many women are therefore recommended to take thyroxine, and it is important to state that this is a life-saving drug. However, we are always more interested in why the thyroid was struggling in the first place, and that leads us back to blood sugars and stress.

Thymus gland: The thymus is part of our immune system. It makes white blood cells called T cells which help fight infection. Commonly, people experience immune issues in the presence of constant stress.

Pancreas: We heard a bit about the pancreas earlier when we were talking about blood sugars. The pancreas has two main functions: most of its work is supposed to be supporting digestion by producing digestive enzymes to break down food. However, we know that it is also responsible for producing insulin and glucagon to regulate blood sugars.

Adrenal glands: The adrenals are entirely responsible for making our stress hormones. But they also make about 35 per cent of sex hormones and almost 50 per cent of post-menopausal sex hormones, so stress and adrenal function profoundly affect hormonal balance. The adrenals also make a hormone called aldosterone, which plays a central role in the regulation of blood pressure and fluid regulation such as sweating, saliva, and in our colon. Aldosterone is less talked about than the stress hormone cortisol, but the key point to take away here is that high blood pressure and water retention (which are commonly medicated) are historically considered to be to do with heart issues and kidneys respectively, but they can in fact be to do with overworked adrenal glands, which brings the focus back to why the adrenals are overworking.

Testicles (male)/ovaries (female): These glands make and secrete our sex hormones: testosterone for males and oestrogen/progesterone as well as testosterone for females. In men, the testes also produce sperm, and in females, the ovaries store and release eggs at ovulation. Because of the connection with the adrenal glands' production of sex hormones, and their dependency on the production of hormones by other glands such as the thyroid, the testes and ovaries can have inhibited function during times of stress.

In simplistic terms, our stress response happens when the hypothalamus and pituitary gland believe we are in danger, either from something outside of us, such as a fire, or from something inside of us, like our blood sugars dropping dangerously low; they will communicate with the adrenal glands using messenger hormones that signal the need for adrenaline and cortisol, our stress hormones, to be produced. Once the adrenal glands have produced adrenaline and cortisol, there is another message sent back to the hypothalamus and pituitary gland – again, via hormones – signalling that this has been done. This return message is called a *negative feedback loop*.

This whole communication is called the *HPA axis* (hypothalamic–pituitary–adrenal axis)

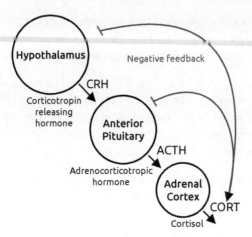

DIAGRAM 6 – THE HPA AXIS

The problem for our hypothalamus and pituitary gland in today's world is that because of our constant exposure to the stressors we explored earlier, they perceive we are under constant threat. This perception means that the pituitary gland ignores the negative feedback loop and continues to send "stress memos", which eventually leads to the feedback loop communication breaking down. This breakdown is called HPA dysregulation.

We've mentioned adrenaline and cortisol a few times, and these hormones are often mentioned in the media, but why are they important?

Both adrenaline and cortisol are made in our adrenal glands in response to stress.

Adrenaline is only released when a threat is perceived. Its job is fast action; it increases your heart rate and blood pressure and boosts your energy – when we have adrenaline in our bloodstream, we feel more alert, have more energy, are less sensitive to pain, and have heightened senses and increased breathing. It is literally getting you ready to fight or take flight.

Cortisol then takes over to clean up the mess left in adrenaline's wake. It is anti-inflammatory, immunosuppressive, and improves stress tolerance. Cortisol's function in this instance is twofold. First, it releases glucose to give you enough energy to deal with the stressor until it has passed. Second, it sends a signal to your brain to lower the level of the acute stress response.

All that sounds great, and it is in small bursts, but if we are in a constant state of "perceived threat" with elevated blood sugars and reduced digestion, we are in for trouble in the long term.

The endocrine system is supposed to work a bit like an orchestra. Each of the glands plays a part, and when they play together properly, a symphony is created. This translates to humans as feeling well, being energized, and having good immunity.

However, if one or two of the glands are playing too loudly or behaving in a diva-like fashion, the orchestra can't play properly. We end up with a noisy mess – or, in human health terms, we end up with a stack of symptoms. If the adrenals are struggling due to high levels of stress, we can see the rest of the endocrine system, including the ovaries, also starting to struggle. So you can see the importance of dealing with stress, especially at times of hormonal transition such as perimenopause.

Common signs of a stressed endocrine system are:

- feeling tired and wired
- insomnia
- anxiety
- menstrual symptoms
- low libido
- depression
- digestive complaints including IBS
- faintness and dizziness
- weakness
- fatigue
- heart palpitations
- emotional hypersensitivity
- headaches and general unexplained body aches
- lower back pain
- sensitive skin
- nausea, diarrhoea, and vomiting
- abdominal pain and bloating
- food cravings
- clumsiness and confusion.

And if we are in this constant state of threat, our orchestra isn't playing nicely together. Our adrenals are taking centre stage and not letting anyone else be heard.

As with insulin resistance and leptin resistance, when we have too much cortisol flooding the body, our cells become resistant to it. It's common, therefore, for the other glands to start to overwork just to be heard.

Thyroid issues are common in women, and autoimmune disease, which predominantly affects women, is connected to this endocrine dysregulation. In fact, when you look at the list of symptoms above, you can start to identify many, many conditions which we regularly see women medicated for.

The adrenal fatigue myth

There is a myth that the adrenals get burned out or fatigued. It's a myth we ourselves propagated and language we bandied about over the years until we learned better.

It is better to use the term "cortisol dysfunction".

In many people who experience fatigue disorders such as ME, long COVID, chronic fatigue, or fibromyalgia, functional cortisol tests can often show that cortisol is low, not high. It was therefore believed that the adrenals had become burned out and couldn't make any more cortisol. This is not true.

Recent research looks at the fact that the body is not producing cortisol on purpose, because it is anti-inflammatory. The theory is that the immune system wants to stimulate inflammation because it is trying to rid the body of something. This could be:

- a viral infection

- toxic overload

- leptin resistance or sensitivity (imbalanced blood sugars)

- prolonged stress, which creates an environment that depletes immune function.

The question is then, which of these is relevant for the individual? And if it's because of an infection, why isn't the immune system dealing with the infection? And where is the infection or toxic overload coming from?

That is, in the simplest of terms, what is happening in response to stress in the endocrine system, but the impact of stress doesn't stop there. The nervous system is so closely connected to the endocrine system that it will also be in a state of high alert.

Let's look at what that means.

The nervous system and stress

The central nervous system consists of the brain, spinal cord, and all the nerves within our body. Our *autonomic* nervous system is the part of the central nervous system that regulates our involuntary body functions.

The autonomic nervous system has two sides: the *sympathetic* nervous system and the *parasympathetic* nervous system. Both sides control the same parts of the body and the same body functions, but with opposite effect.

The sympathetic nervous system is for "get up and go". When we perceive a threat or are stressed, our sympathetic nervous system kicks into gear and increases heart rate, elevates blood pressure, heightens awareness, elevates respiratory rate, and increases sweating.

The parasympathetic nervous system is for "rest and digest". It works to slow down and bring about a state of calm to the body, allowing it to rest, relax, and repair itself. Parasympathetic responses include an increase of digestive enzymes, decreased heart rate, vaginal dilation, and more relaxed muscles.

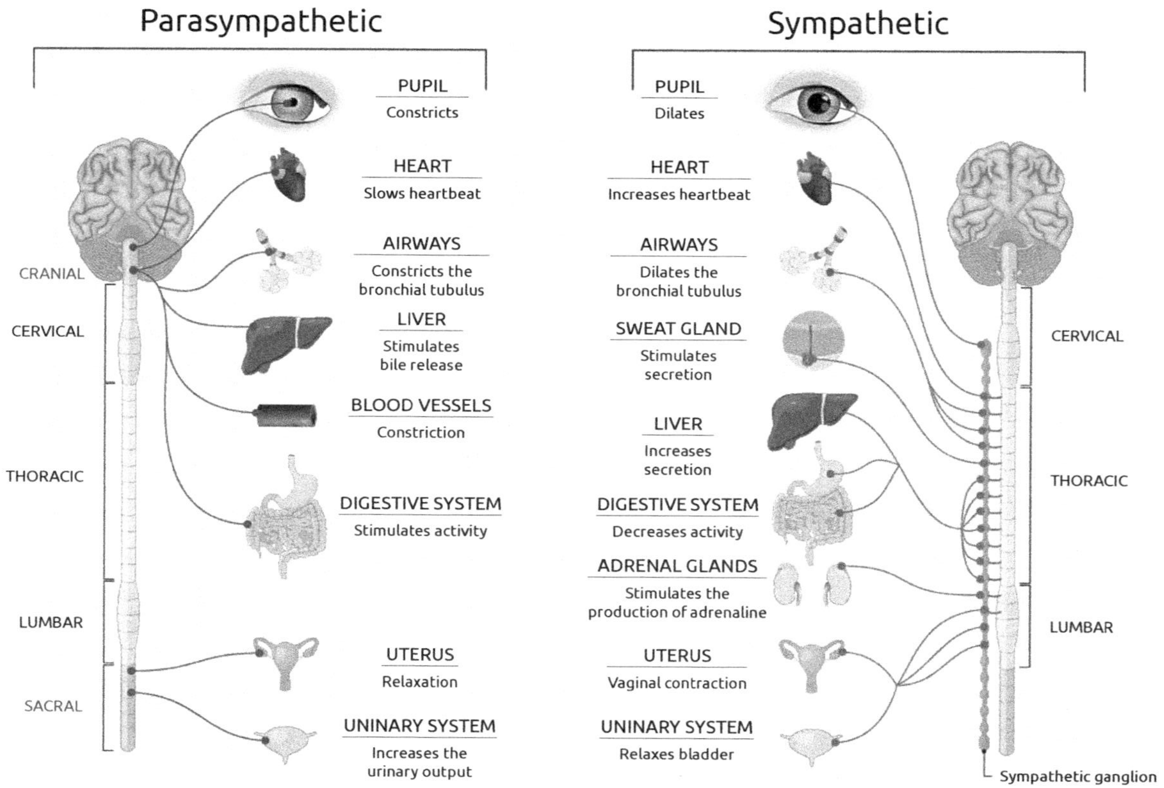

Parasympathetic

PUPIL
Constricts

HEART
Slows heartbeat

AIRWAYS
Constricts the bronchial tubulus

LIVER
Stimulates bile release

BLOOD VESSELS
Constriction

DIGESTIVE SYSTEM
Stimulates activity

UTERUS
Relaxation

UNINARY SYSTEM
Increases the urinary output

CRANIAL

CERVICAL

THORACIC

LUMBAR

SACRAL

Sympathetic

PUPIL
Dilates

HEART
Increases heartbeat

AIRWAYS
Dilates the bronchial tubulus

SWEAT GLAND
Stimulates secretion

LIVER
Increases secretion

DIGESTIVE SYSTEM
Decreases activity

ADRENAL GLANDS
Stimulates the production of adrenaline

UTERUS
Vaginal contraction

UNINARY SYSTEM
Relaxes bladder

CERVICAL

THORACIC

LUMBAR

Sympathetic ganglion

DIAGRAM 7 – THE NERVOUS SYSTEM

The sympathetic nervous system is stimulated in response to adrenaline and cortisol, when it is activated, it shuts down the activity of the parasympathetic nervous system. The prolonged exposure to cortisol, adrenaline, and stress in modern life means that we can spend a lot of time with our parasympathetic nervous system shut down.

We call this being *sympathetic nervous system dominant*, and this state will keep the body in a catch-22: being on high alert triggers more stress hormone, and more stress hormone triggers the sympathetic nervous system to be dominant.

Both the sympathetic and parasympathetic nervous systems are vital to our health and survival. However, for our bodies to live with optimal health and proper function for as long as possible, there must be a balance between the two. If there is a miscommunication between your brain and the impulses that promote sympathetic responses, your body will be functioning in fight-or-flight mode far too often and for far too long, and this can be a major contributing factor to the underlying reasons why women are experiencing an awful menopause.

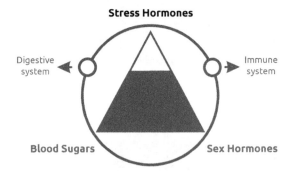

DIAGRAM 8 – THE TRIANGLE OF HORMONAL HEALTH AND STRESS

Stress hormones are a key pillar of the Triangle of Hormonal Health because they have direct interaction with the other two pillars – sex hormones and blood sugars – and the "victims" – digestive and immune function.

Blood sugars

You already know from the previous chapter that the stress hormone cortisol spikes blood sugars and creates insulin imbalances that have knock-on effects with the other blood sugar hormones and symptoms such as anxiety.

Sex hormones

Because it is more important to get out of danger than reproduce, the endocrine system will prioritize the stress response over making our sex hormone progesterone, which we will be exploring in the next chapter.

Digestive function

Because cortisol aids in moving blood flow towards the brain, large muscles, and limbs, and away from the digestive tract, our ability to digest reduces. We already know that being in a stress response creates a situation where we are sympathetic nervous system dominant and have a stimulated vagus nerve. In this state, we stop making digestive acid and enzymes, further impeding our ability to digest.

Immune function

Adrenaline switches on the immune system and promotes an inflammatory response. Cortisol has an anti-inflammatory action; however, in excess quantities it has an inflammatory effect.

> **TAKE-HOME MESSAGE**
>
> The stress response is hugely impactful on every aspect of our health and wellbeing. Stress and poor diet are the two main contributors to the issues we are seeing with human health globally. We must address them. Certainly, there are many aspects of stress that we can't control, but we need to free up bandwidth by reducing exposure to the stressors we can control.
>
> Most women tell us that it isn't possible to remove or reduce any stress, but one of the repeated messages we have received when working with clients with life-affecting perimenopause is that it's amazing what you choose to stop stressing about and rushing around for when your health demands it. The question therefore is: how do we make the choice to reduces stress for our wellbeing before a major illness or condition takes that choice away?

So, that's stress. Now let's get stuck into what is going on with our sex hormones and how all of this affects our menopause!

— CHAPTER 6 —

Sex hormones

And here we are – finally – at the chapter about sex hormones! We hope that on the way to getting to this chapter you've seen why we start with the foundational information – because of how impactive the other hormones are on our sex hormones and vice versa.

During the menopause transition, our hormones are all over the place, and the knock-on effect is profound. The symptoms we looked at earlier are so often skimmed over that women are commonly taken by surprise by how impactive this transition is.

Before we look at what is happening during perimenopause to post-menopause, let's talk about what was happening during our monthly cycles before the hormonal turbulence began, so that we can understand more deeply what is causing us the issues during menopause.

Women have three sex hormones: oestrogen, progesterone, and testosterone.

It's important to know what they are and what they do, so we can begin to identify our symptoms based on what is happening with each of them.

Let's start with oestrogen.

Oestrogen

Oestrogen (also often shown as estrogen) is made in the ovaries, fat cells, and adrenal glands; there are oestrogen receptors in every single part of the body including the brain, bowel, thyroid gland, and muscle. At puberty, oestrogen plays a role in the development of the secondary sex characteristics (such as breast growth, menstrual cycle, and body hair development). It is also responsible for thickening the endometrial lining and regulating the menstrual cycle.

It is an "excitor" hormone and stimulates the body.

Oestrogen is an umbrella term for three different hormones:

- oestradiol (also often shown as estradiol) – the predominant fertility hormone

- oestriol (also often shown as estriol) – the pregnancy version of oestrogen

- oestrone (also often shown as estrone) – the hormone present post-menopause after oestradiol stops being made.

Oestrogen is used by the body and then broken down by the liver and excreted. It is important to note that perimenopausal women can have oestrogen levels 20–30 per cent higher than those of women of reproductive age before perimenopause, due to the fluctuations in hormones at this time.

Oestrogen plays many vital roles in the body when there is the correct amount. It:

- regulates body fat

- promotes female reproduction function

- promotes heart health

- promotes bone formation and cell health

- regulates blood sugars.

Not enough oestrogen in post-menopause can cause the following symptoms:

- mood swings

- weight gain or loss

- memory loss

- menstrual cycle cessation

- vaginal dryness

- irritability

- fatigue

- hot flushes

- insomnia

- stress and anxiety

- loss of bone density

- reduced muscle mass

- increased potential for stroke and heart attack.

There are two other types of oestrogen that have a profound effect on women's bodies: phyto-oestrogens and xeno-oestrogens.

Phyto-oestrogens
These are plant chemicals that have a similar effect on our body as oestrogen. These can be very beneficial in supporting women through the latter stages of menopause, but they can wreak havoc earlier in life if we are exposed to them a lot, and they can mess up our natural hormone signaling.

Xeno-oestrogens
Xeno-oestrogens (pronounced "zeeno-oestrogens") are compounds that mimic oestrogen, and they commonly contribute to health issues. Xeno means "foreign". They are also referred to as endocrine-disrupting chemicals (EDCs).

They are fake oestrogens brought about by pollution, toxicity, poor diet, and an imbalanced gut microbiome. Xeno-oestrogens can disturb our natural oestrogen levels and cause a build-up which the body struggles to process. Historically high exposure to xeno-oestrogens can be a reason why women feel so awful during perimenopause and can be a major factor contributing to why women aren't able to tolerate or process HRT. They are also a contributor to many hormone issues earlier in life.

Xeno-oestrogens are therefore a major contributor to having too much oestrogen.

Having too much oestrogen is common. This is called oestrogen dominance.

What do we really mean by oestrogen dominance?

Oestrogen dominance
Oestrogen dominance causes huge issues in the body. We commonly see a pattern of symptoms suggesting women are oestrogen dominant throughout their whole lives.

Oestrogen dominance symptoms include a variety of conditions that women can have experienced historically, but which are also common during perimenopause. These include:

- heavy periods or period issues

- breast pain

- fibroids

- premenstrual irritability

- weight gain

- thyroid suppression and increased risk of breast cancer

- gut dysbiosis and digestive issues

- immune function impairment including histamine issues and allergies

- premenstrual syndrome and premenstrual dysphoric disorder (PMDD)

- polycystic ovary syndrome (PCOS)

- endometriosis

- adenomyosis

- hormone-sensitive cancers.

Oestrogen dominance is a big problem. When in balance, oestrogen helps optimize the action of insulin in reducing blood sugars. However, when there is too much oestrogen, this action is affected, and we are more susceptible to insulin resistance. Equally, when post-menopausal oestrogen is lower, we have an increased susceptibility to insulin resistance. This is one of the reasons for weight gain in perimenopause. The connection between insulin and oestrogen doesn't just happen in women; it also happens in men, and we see in obesity that men are developing the sex characteristics of women such as enlarged breasts and hips. We are therefore seeing the interaction between insulin and oestrogen become one of the major health issues in the world.

Causes of oestrogen dominance

Many things trigger oestrogen dominance, such as hormonal birth control, impaired gut function, perimenopause, hyperinsulinemia, stress, xeno-oestrogens, endocrine disruptor chemical exposure, and HPA axis dysregulation. This list shows how women could have been dealing with oestrogen dominance for many years.

> ## TAKE-HOME MESSAGE
> Oestrogen is an exciter hormone, and we need it in the right amount to be well. Too much of it can cause all sorts of issues in the body, as well as too little. Because of the effect of xeno-oestrogens, our body can act as though it has too much of it, even if it doesn't.

Oestrogen dominance can also occur when oestrogen levels are optimal but we have less than optimal levels of progesterone. As we will discover, this is something that happens in perimenopause, but we are also seeing it in younger and younger girls, often in their early teens.

Let's have a look at why we want enough of the magical hormone that is progesterone.

Progesterone

Primarily, progesterone helps prepare the female body for conception and pregnancy while regulating the menstrual cycle. It is made from a hormone called pregnenolone (this information will become important later).

Progesterone is a startlingly beneficial hormone; it is produced in large quantities by the ovaries during ovulation. It helps prepare the lining of the uterus to receive the egg if a sperm fertilizes it. It also acts on the breasts, brain, immune system, and detoxification system. It is also a calming hormone, as opposed to oestrogen which is an exciter hormone.

Some of the benefits of progesterone include the following:

- **It boosts energy** by stimulating the thyroid and heating up the metabolism. This is why body temperature goes up half a degree when progesterone is made after ovulation. It also stabilizes communication between the hypothalamus and adrenal glands, and so relieves HPA dysregulation, which we explored in the previous chapter.

- **It calms us down.** Progesterone is a natural calming hormone.

- **It soothes mood and rescues sleep** (remember this when we look at what happens to hormones during menopause later on in this chapter).

- **It nourishes hair and clears skin.**

- **It lightens periods** by counteracting oestrogen's stimulating effect on the uterine lining.

- **It prevents autoimmune disease** because it modulates immune function, reduces inflammation, and upregulates detoxification enzymes.

- **It builds bones and muscle** by stimulating bone-building cells and the growth of new muscle.

- **It protects against some cancers** by counteracting oestrogen's stimulating effect on breast and uterine tissue.

- **It helps to regulate insulin.** It controls and stabilizes the production of insulin in the pancreas, which, given the worldwide issue of insulin resistance, is a very important job.

Conditions associated with progesterone deficiency include:

- PCOS
- heavy periods
- fibroids
- acne
- hair loss
- endometriosis
- autoimmune disease
- insomnia
- inflammation
- forgetfulness
- lack of concentration
- "wired but tired"

- depression
- IBS
- excess insulin production, leading to premenstrual syndrome (PMS)
- premenstrual migraines
- infertility
- perimenopause
- menopause
- osteoporosis
- primary ovarian failure
- anxiety
- bloating
- irregular periods
- palpitations with no cause found in the heart
- short luteal phase (the time between ovulation and your period, which should be at least 11 days)
- low temperatures in the luteal phase
- premenstrual spotting.

Progesterone is vital to women's physical and mental health because of its calming action, and it is this fact that is often overlooked by the medical model, which focuses more on oestrogen levels.

We are going to be looking at this in more depth, but the fact is that, in many circles, progesterone has been wrongly reduced to just being important for pregnancy. Its effects on digestion, emotions, the nervous system, mood, weight stabilization, and sleep are often sidelined.

When we look at the history of women's healthcare in the developed world, it is fascinating to view many of the conditions that women have been labelled with, such as "hysteria", through the lens of a lack of progesterone. It becomes incredibly frustrating when you realize that many conditions such as PMDD have links to low progesterone but haven't been treated with progesterone.

In fact, there is some fascinating research emerging about the use of natural progesterone with conditions such as autoimmune disease and endometriosis due to its anti-inflammatory action.[1]

We will be diving into this topic more deeply when we explore HRT.

When googling "too much progesterone", there is a standard list of symptoms:

- tenderness in the breasts
- rapidly changing moods
- anxiety
- feeling depressed
- being bloated
- lack of sex drive
- fatigue
- drowsiness
- muscle weakness.

What we can't establish is how women have too much progesterone, apart from the rare case of an adrenal disease or if they have been using contraceptives or HRT. Our theory from personal and clinical experience is that most women have too little, and often from early on in their life. We will be exploring why this is later in this chapter. The "too much" progesterone discussed here could well be due to synthetic progesterone. Much has been published about the links between sleep disorders and menopause, given that progesterone has a sedative as well as anxiety-reducing effect.[2]

> **TAKE-HOME MESSAGE**
> The important thing to take from this is that progesterone is our only *calming* hormone. It helps sleep and stabilizes our mood and weight. This is going to be important later. In fact, it's probably the most important point in this book.

But what about testosterone?

Testosterone

Testosterone is commonly known as the male hormone, but women produce it as well.

In women, it boosts:

- sex drive
- mood and confidence
- memory and concentration
- ligaments, muscle, and bone.

Historically, testosterone has been considered less important for women, but any menopausal woman who's trying to carry on working and having a semblance of a normal life will tell you that testosterone replacement therapy can be a game changer for women struggling with low energy, low libido, and apathy. It is currently not licensed for female use in the UK, but some doctors are nevertheless prescribing it.

Testosterone is made in the adrenal glands and the ovaries, and plays a role in the menstrual cycle. It is interesting to note here that the ovaries are highly sensitive to insulin. In the presence of too much insulin, the ovaries will produce testosterone, which can then lead to PCOS.

Testosterone can become too high sometimes due to an insulin imbalance and having a high percentage of fat cells in the body. This causes the ovaries to create more testosterone.

Too much testosterone can cause:

- skin issues such as acne
- excess hair or baldness
- fatigue
- anxiety and depression
- weight gain
- period irregularity
- low sex drive
- fertility issues
- PCOS
- suppressed immune system.

Low testosterone can cause:

- lack of libido
- low mood
- low energy and drive
- reduced muscle mass.

> **TAKE-HOME MESSAGE**
> Women also have testosterone but in smaller amounts than men. It is essential for our "get up and go"!

Now that we have a better understanding of our hormones, let's have a look at how they are supposed to work together in a healthy monthly cycle.

What happens during the menstrual cycle?

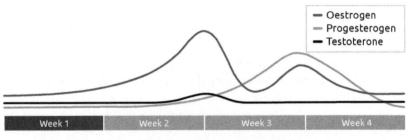

DIAGRAM 9 – THE FEMALE MONTHLY CYCLE

The female menstrual cycle lasts between 21 days and 35 days (the average being 28 days) and prepares the female body for a possible pregnancy.

The follicular phase
The follicular stage starts on the first day of our bleed (day 1) as we shed the previous month's lining (if there's no pregnancy). This stage lasts 3–7 days.

The hypothalamus releases a hormone (GnRH) which tells the pituitary to produce follicle-stimulating hormone (FSH); this starts the ovulation process.

FSH stimulates the development of immature eggs in the follicles of the ovaries, which is why this is called the follicular phase. Each month, the ovaries take it in turns to release an egg.

At this stage, the follicles have started producing oestrogen which thickens the endometrium (womb lining) in preparation for a possible fertilized egg.

Ovulation

Ovulation starts in the second week, around day 14, and is the shortest phase, lasting 2–4 days. This is when a woman is most fertile.

There is a rise in testosterone as the body heads towards ovulation because testosterone boosts a woman's sex drive.

The follicles continue to produce oestrogen, and the womb lining continues to thicken. Around ovulation, there is a spike in oestrogen to optimize the chance of fertilization. Oestrogen changes the mucus, making it more hospitable for sperm. And a peak of oestrogen signals to the pituitary gland to release luteinizing hormone (LH) which, with FSH, pushes ovulation to happen. This is known as the LH surge.

The egg is released by the follicle and enters the fallopian tube where it will survive for 12–24 hours. If it isn't fertilized, the egg is reabsorbed by the body or excreted in the next period.

If fertilization occurs, the woman will start producing human chorionic gonadotrophin, which is the hormone picked up on pregnancy tests. This hormone is produced by the embryo and signals to the corpus luteum to keep making oestrogen and progesterone to maintain the pregnancy.

The corpus luteum is a hormone-secreting structure made from the remains of the follicle. Its primary purpose is to pulse out hormones, and it is essential for conception and for the pregnancy to last.

The luteal phase

The luteal phase lasts 10–16 days and always precedes menstruation by 14 days.

The corpus luteum starts to produce progesterone, preventing the release of another egg for the rest of the cycle. It also signals to the pituitary to stop producing FSH, which results in oestrogen levels falling. Progesterone then surpasses oestrogen as the dominant hormone, and the rise in progesterone acts as a feedback loop to the pituitary gland so that LH and FSH continue to fall.

The corpus luteum becomes the corpus albicans, which doesn't release hormones, so the level of oestrogen and progesterone start to decrease, leading to menstruation.

TAKE-HOME MESSAGE
Oestrogen and testosterone peak around ovulation and then reduce, and progesterone peaks around the week before our bleed.

It's interesting to note that many women have symptoms around ovulation. Symptoms such as ovulation pain (which is technically called *Mittelschmerz*, German for "middle pain"), headaches and migraines, bloating and IBS, PMDD and premenstrual tension (PMT) often start or peak around ovulation.

Medically, these symptoms are put down to hormone imbalance, which is rather vague. We have always been interested in *which hormones* are imbalanced.

Oestrogen deficiency only happens due to some rare conditions or menopause, so it is commonly not enough progesterone causing the issues. This is referred to as "oestrogen dominance". We are going to discuss this further when we drill into what happens during the menopause, but the key thing to remember is that it is happening much earlier in women's lives than menopause, and it is overlooked.

When looking online, it's very easy to find references to high or low oestrogen, progesterone, or testosterone, and when we find that a hormone is high or low, the focus becomes fixing that specific issue, not looking at why the hormones are imbalanced.

But the "why" is more useful when trying to understand our health. Hormones fluctuate and they work like a seesaw – too much of this will make it look as though there is too little of that, and vice versa – but when we start trying to figure out why the body is in this state of flux, we can get more balance.

The main point to understand here is that *all three of these hormones are essential* for a woman's health and vitality. However, for good health, they need to exist in a delicate balance with each other.

When one is too low, the other acts in an "unopposed" way and issues arise. If one is too high, we don't have enough response from the other lower ones to keep us symptom-free. This delicate balance can be easily destabilized, and this destabilization often happens many, many years before the natural fluctuation at perimenopause.

But what does happen during perimenopause to post-menopause?

Perimenopause, menopause, and premature menopause

Even though women can spend up to 20 years going on the journey from perimenopause through menopause and into post-menopause, we still don't talk about the process transparently. Doctors often miss the symptoms of perimenopause, and women can suffer with the fallout for years before blood tests will show this is what is happening.

Perimenopause

Perimenopause is a period of transition where the ovaries gradually start to produce less hormones. Typically, this starts in a woman's 40s, but it can start much earlier.

The menopause itself is the time during which our bleeds are stopping; confusingly, this is still called perimenopause.

After 12 months of missing a bleed, a woman is considered post-menopausal.

Perimenopause can start up to ten years before a woman becomes "post-menopausal".

The first sign of perimenopause is usually irregular periods. This can mean either missing periods or having them too frequently, having them temporarily regulate, before becoming irregular again. Periods may be heavier than usual or much lighter. Some women taking birth control pills may not experience irregular periods but may notice other symptoms such as unexplained mood changes.

During the last one to two years of perimenopause, oestrogen levels decline at a faster rate, which usually brings on symptoms also experienced by menopausal women. These commonly include:

- hot flushes
- breast tenderness
- lowered libido
- fatigue
- mood swings
- anxiety or depression
- difficulty sleeping
- weight gain
- hair thinning or loss.

The symptoms aren't just physical; there is often huge emotional fallout with perimenopause.

Oestrogen stimulates serotonin, a major mood neurotransmitter that brings on feelings of happiness. When oestrogen levels drop, it can cause a drop in serotonin in the brain, causing feelings of sadness or depression. Oestrogen and progesterone also work to manage production of cortisol, and so feelings of panic, stress, and anxiety may be heightened as these hormone levels change.

Women commonly report lack of confidence and feeling overwhelmed and anxious during perimenopause. Weight gain during menopause is very common.

What long-term health problems are tied to menopause?

The loss of oestrogen linked with post-menopause has been tied to several health problems that become more common as women age. After menopause, women are more likely to have:

- osteoporosis
- heart disease
- poorly working bladder and bowel
- greater risk of Alzheimer's disease
- poor skin elasticity/increased wrinkling
- poor muscle power and tone
- some weakening in vision, such as from cataracts and macular degeneration.

What is happening to hormones during menopause?

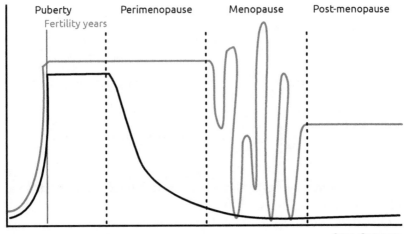

Grey – Oestrogen
Black – Progesterone

DIAGRAM 10 – THE HORMONE PATHWAY FROM PUBERTY TO POST-MENOPAUSE

In this diagram, we are focusing on oestrogen and progesterone. Although testosterone is important to women, we have much less of it, and its menopause trajectory isn't as important to understand as the two primary sex hormones. We will be talking about its importance in Chapter 12 about HRT.

If you look at the graph, you can see that in puberty both progesterone and oestrogen are meant to rise. During our fertile years, when we are experiencing a monthly cycle, they maintain a consistent ratio with oestrogen presenting in slightly higher amounts than progesterone.

Early in the onset of perimenopause, progesterone starts to drop rapidly, but oestrogen maintains its level for quite some time.

Oestrogen levels now start to fluctuate wildly through the menopause transition until they finally drop post-menopause.

Women can experience quite dramatic day-by-day changes, with oestrogen and progesterone levels wildly fluctuating. Sometimes oestrogen may be high, and at other times it may be low, which means it can be very hard to work out what is going on in your body. What we do know is that progesterone will always be low.

According to Dr John Lee, in his book *What Your Doctor May Not Tell You About Menopause*,[3] oestrogen levels "drop only 40 to 60 percent at menopause, while progesterone levels can drop to nearly zero". What we've always questioned is why does the mainstream approach to menopause focus so heavily on oestrogen? If progesterone is the first hormone to significantly reduce during early perimenopause, why is it that oestrogen is tested and used as an indicator of being in perimenopause? Why is oestrogen hormone replacement available over the counter at pharmacies but progesterone is ignored? Why does the medical model favour high doses of oestrogen at a time when oestrogen is already too dominant?

We've never been given a satisfactory answer.

We are going to explore how progesterone is ignored even when women are given HRT in Chapter 12 but for now we want to explain why we believe low progesterone is the better name for oestrogen dominance and why it is a more significant issue in menopause and other hormone-related conditions, such as PMDD, than previously thought.

We've previously looked at the importance of the adrenal glands and how, if we are under stress, they will act like very unhappy "divas" of the endocrine system and pull attention away from the other glands.

Our adrenal glands make a variety of hormones, some of which we explored earlier – remember we talked about aldosterone for blood pressure and fluid balancing. Adrenaline and noradrenaline are transmitters that play an essential role in the stress response – but they don't just deal with stress hormones. They also produce a percentage of our sex hormones. It's not

just our ovaries that make testosterone, oestrogen, and progesterone. Our adrenal glands do too...
Unless we are stressed or have been in contact with a stressor.
If this happens, we will end up in a process called the *pregnenolone steal*.

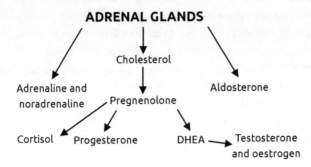

DIAGRAM II – THE PREGNENOLONE STEAL

Looking at the diagram from the top down we see a lot of long words and lines, so let's break it down.

Our adrenal glands use the fat in our diet to make cholesterol.

As an aside, can we just talk about cholesterol, please, because it is very misunderstood and unfairly demonized. We need cholesterol to perform important jobs like making hormones, building cells, helping our metabolism work properly, producing digestive bile acids, and healing inflammation in the body. It is not the bad guy it is made out to be! We love and need cholesterol!

When we experience inflammation in our arteries, for example, our body sends cholesterol to act like Polyfilla to calm and mend the microscopic tears caused by the expansion of the inflammation. Where does the inflammation that leads to systematically high cholesterol originate? Diet, gut issues, food intolerances, stress, and hormone imbalances are usually the culprits. It makes little sense to blame cholesterol for all the inflammation created by our toxic lifestyles and to take medication to reduce cholesterol and not understand where the actual problem is.

But back to the process of making hormones in the adrenal glands.

Your liver makes cholesterol out of the fat you eat, which is one of the reasons eating high-quality fat is so important. From the cholesterol, we make a chain of hormones called steroid hormones. We often know of the word "steroids" from the medical use of synthetic cortisol derivatives to reduce inflammation (these medications are called corticosteroids) or the steroids used for athletic enhancement (synthetic forms of testosterone). Our steroid hormones include cortisol, oestrogen, progesterone, and testosterone.

Here is how the chain works.

Cholesterol makes a precursor hormone called pregnenolone. Pregnenolone itself has lots of great characteristics including antidepressant properties, improvement of memory and cognitive functions, control of pain and stress, and relieving symptoms of mood disorder. But it is also called the "mother hormone" because it makes hormones from itself.

On the right side of the diagram, we see pregnenolone making another precursor hormone called DHEA. DHEA also has many benefits. It's called the "anti-ageing" hormone, and it can be beneficial for depression, osteoporosis, and vaginal atrophy.

DHEA makes oestrogen and testosterone.

Looking at the left-hand branch, we can see that pregnenolone makes progesterone, and all would be well if that was the end of this story. But it isn't, and here's the rub – if we are under stress, the body chooses to make cortisol instead of make cortisol instead of progesterone – it doesn't turn it. This is because it is more important for us to have the fuel to run away from danger than to be calm and have the right environment to hold a baby in our womb or sleep. Getting away from danger is the priority.

If we are under stress, progesterone is not made and instead we make cortisol.

The problem, as we've explored previously, is that our body cannot distinguish between a non-vital threat and a vital one, and we are surrounded by non-vital threats, so the choice to make cortisol over progesterone is happening commonly. With that in mind, let's revisit some concepts we discussed previously and paint this picture more vividly.

When we prioritize cortisol over progesterone, we have no capability to wind down. We will experience anxiety, mood destabilization, and unstable blood sugars. Our HPA axis will be dysregulated, which creates a catch-22 situation: more cortisol = less progesterone = increased stress = less progesterone production = more cortisol.

This cortisol will signal that we need to be in the sympathetic nervous system response and, again, contribute to being a stressor that ensures even less progesterone is created.

If we are making less progesterone, it stands to reason that our oestrogen will be higher, and testosterone might also be higher in relation to progesterone. Even if the levels of these hormones show to be "normal" on a blood test, what we see is that they are "unopposed" if progesterone production is reduced. These hormones require a delicate balance like a seesaw, and if one is lower, we can display symptoms as if the others were too high.

The question really is how important this is, as we are only talking about the progesterone made by the adrenals. The answer is we don't really know.

In rats, the adrenal glands make 70 per cent of the progesterone used by the body. The answer we got when we asked an endocrinologist was that in humans the adrenal glands make only 2 per cent of the progesterone. Wikipedia gives a figure of around 10 per cent, and other references we have found and quoted previously say 35 per cent.

It is frustrating to not be able to get a proper answer because we believe this information is the missing link as to why we are seeing symptoms suggesting a lack of progesterone in women of all ages, including puberty.

The situation with the pregnenolone steal can also happen when we aren't able to make enough pregnenolone. This would happen because of (a) not eating enough fat and (b) stress. So yep, basically all women who have grown up with the low-fat diet craze and have to navigate the modern life craze would be at risk of this issue. It is this low progesterone issue, compounded by the issues we have discussed in the previous chapters, that we feel is the reason why modern menopause is so life-affecting for many women.

Although the focus of this book is menopause, we want to highlight that the issue of the body prioritizing cortisol over progesterone isn't just happening in menopause. It's happening our whole lives. Many of the symptoms we see in clinic (and have experienced ourselves) are, in fact, signs of low progesterone: any period issues such as heavy or inconsistent periods, PMT, endometriosis, PNDD, androgen-excessive PCOS – and there are even implications that fatigue disorders such as a chronic fatigue/ME or even autoimmune conditions can be contributed to by a reduction in progesterone. Young women who are struggling with weight and periods can be shown to have low progesterone when they have blood tests done by the GP. Most practitioners use the phrase "oestrogen dominance", but blood tests commonly show that oestrogen levels are "normal" but progesterone is low.

Without progesterone, women really can feel as though they are going insane: we will be snappy, intolerant, unable to sleep, anxious, have poor digestion – the list is endless. Medically, it seems that progesterone hasn't been recognized for its effect on both our physical wellbeing and mental wellbeing, and there is a belief that synthetic progesterone does the same job as natural progesterone (it doesn't, as we will discuss later).

TAKE-HOME MESSAGE

Progesterone is reduced in response to stress, and it drops much, much earlier than oestrogen. Rebalancing this essential hormone can make the menopause transition smoother.

Understanding this and ensuring that we are given the right hormones during menopause are essential.

The Triangle of Hormonal Health and how it is affected by sex hormones

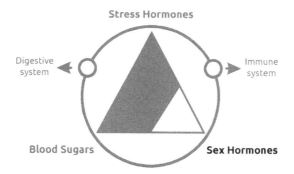

DIAGRAM 12 – THE TRIANGLE OF HORMONAL HEALTH FOCUSING ON SEX HORMONES

Sex hormones are the third key pillar of the Triangle of Hormonal Health, and imbalances here have a big knock-on effect on the other hormone systems and our digestion and immune system.

Of course, in menopause our triangle is going to be imbalanced because the sex hormones are fluctuating as part of this natural transition. It is imperative therefore to create stability in the other legs. It is because women today have poor diets and/or stressful lifestyles that menopause is so challenging.

Let's look at a summary of what is happening throughout the rest of the triangle through the lens of destabilized progesterone and oestrogen.

Blood sugars

Oestrogen and progesterone affect how cells respond to insulin. High oestrogen and low progesterone increase insulin resistance, resulting in weight gain and inflammation.

Conversely, later in menopause, low oestrogen can also cause impaired insulin action.

Glucose and insulin spikes disrupt ovulation and prevent our hormones from triggering ovulation and the creation of progesterone arising from ovulation. Without ovulation, you cannot produce progesterone, which leads to oestrogen dominance.

Our fat cells secrete oestrogen. The more sugar eaten, the more fat cells are created, and, in turn, the more oestrogen they secrete. This oestrogen adds to the oestrogen your endocrine system produces.

Stress

Circulating oestrogen (such as xeno-oestrogens or non-metabolized oestrogen) can increase cortisol levels.

High cortisol reduces progesterone production.

Chronic stress can affect testosterone production, resulting in a decline in sex drive.

Digestive function

Too much oestrogen wreaks havoc on our digestive tract by causing gut dysbiosis.

Too much oestrogen can cause issues with movement of food through the gut.

Immune function

Excess oestrogen, xeno-oestrogens, and lowered progesterone change our immune response and can contribute to immune issues.

TAKE-HOME MESSAGE

- Low progesterone = high oestrogen = insulin resistance.

- Low progesterone = high cortisol = increased HPA axis dysregulation.

- Increased HPA axis dysregulation = increased likelihood of being in the sympathetic nervous system dominant response.

- Increased sympathetic nervous system = lowered progesterone.

How do I know if I have low or high oestrogen and progesterone?

This is where it gets a bit tricky.

When we are going through menopause, the symptoms of low oestrogen can be the same as high oestrogen, so it's not always clear. We can try to take an educated guess, but there are some clues.

First, it is useful to have an idea of where you are in your menopause. If you are still bleeding regularly, it's more likely that you are in the perimenopause transition where you have low progesterone, but your oestrogen is either comparatively high or starting to fluctuate.

Once your periods start to become irregular, then it can be even more of a guessing game. Ultimately, by this point, it doesn't matter too much, as we will be applying the solutions that we talk about in Part Two of this book.

So, this is in no way an exact science, just a way to help you assess what might be happening in your body.

If you are still bleeding regularly and you experience some of the following:

- sore breasts
- weight gain
- insomnia
- palpitations
- spotting
- feeling "wired but tired"
- anxiety
- digestive upsets

- mood swings
- allergies or food intolerances
- skin issues
- changes in sexual desire
- autoimmunity
- body odour
- changes in appetite (either increase or decrease)...

...these can be signs that your oestrogen is high and progesterone is low.

If your periods have become irregular or scanty and you experience some of the following:

- low mood (life feels colourless)
- exhausted
- no joy

- vaginal dryness
- spotting...

...these could be signs that your progesterone and oestrogen are low.

Hot flushes are a good metric.

Quick, violent hot flushes that come on quickly with no warning and are finished in less than two minutes are a sign of low progesterone (you are having a rush of cortisol and adrenaline). They are often accompanied by a palpitation or a tummy flip caused by the adrenaline.

Very slow hot flushes that go on for around ten minutes, radiate from somewhere inside (commonly the chest or behind the knee), spread slowly throughout the rest of your body, and leave you feeling roasting hot (and even heat the furniture around you) are a sign of low oestrogen.

Experiencing a mix of both types would show that both hormones are low; this is more common as we are going through the part of menopause where we are missing bleeds (but it can still happen earlier).

It can be a bit of a guessing game, but rather than get frustrated (easier said than done), we recommend observing and making notes and looking for trends. Menopause can really require some patience!

What happens when we go to the doctors?

While many areas of the NHS are exemplary, the state of women's healthcare is shocking. Literally shocking. Sadly, this is often highlighted during menopause.

GPs are often at a loss about the right course of action because menopause training isn't mandatory, so it is a bit of a postcode lottery as to whether you receive good advice.

If you are over the age of 45, the NHS won't give you blood tests because it is presupposed that your hormones are unstable and there is no point testing. Instead, you will be offered HRT. We are going to talk about the different options in Part Two, so you know what to ask for.

If you are below 40, you will usually be considered too young to be perimenopausal, and unless you are in the surgery repeatedly or have private medical insurance so you can ask to see an endocrinologist, it is likely that you will be given antidepressants. These medications are common because many women are talking about mood swings or anxiety.

If you are between the age of 40 and 45, you might be offered a blood test or will be allowed one if you request one.

Medically, perimenopause can be proven only when your body has had a sharp rise in FSH (follicle-stimulating hormone) and LH (luteinizing hormone). These hormones signal to the ovaries that it's time to ovulate (stimulate the ovum follicle), and during menopause, when the ability for the body to ovulate diminishes, we produce more and more of them. An analogy would be that the hormones are knocking on the door of the ovaries to get them to do what they are meant to do, but during menopause the ovaries have stopped hearing the knock, so more FSH is sent to knock repeatedly... meaning we have high levels of FSH and LH.

It is more common for oestrogen to be tested, but when you see what is happening in early perimenopause, that doesn't make sense. It is uncommon for progesterone to be tested, which is why a lot of early perimenopause can be missed in blood tests and women are told their results are "normal". Until FSH and LH become elevated, which can happen quite far into perimenopause, we don't see the true picture.

If the GP is prepared to do a hormone blood test, ask them to check your progesterone levels. It will be a snapshot of your progesterone which rises and falls, so it is not the complete picture, but it will give you an indication of what level of progesterone is present.

TAKE-HOME MESSAGE

Too much oestrogen is actually too little progesterone.

Too much testosterone is actually too little progesterone.

Too little progesterone is usually caused by stress.

Let's move on to digestion and the immune system as the knock-on effects of this hormonal fallout are huge!

— CHAPTER 7 —

Digestive function

Why are we talking about digestion?

The gut microbiome and digestion are systemically overlooked in menopause care by the medical model. Bearing in mind that many women are entering menopause with a history of irritable bowel syndrome, constipation, or an inflammatory bowel disease such as Crohn's, gut health is essential to talk about; repeatedly, however, we have seen celebrities, high-profile doctors, and menopause experts overlooking this important piece of the picture.

Although some women say HRT is a "silver bullet", millions of others still struggle with debilitating symptoms despite taking HRT.

There are multiple reasons why this could be the case, but we commonly see the following:

- Women have been given too much oestrogen too early in perimenopause when they are oestrogen dominant.

- They have been given synthetic progesterone when they really needed natural progesterone.

- They do not have good gut health and therefore either cannot absorb the hormones (typically in this case, we see that they have historically had "absorption" issues and have regularly needed to take iron or vitamin B12).

- They are intolerant to the ingredients in the hormone medication (such as peanut or soy).

We are deep-diving into HRT in Part Two, but we wanted to bring the connection here so we can start to explore what gut health really means and recognize that good gut health is essential to feeling good during menopause. Actually, good gut health is essential to feeling good throughout our whole lives!

Menopause often shines a light on issues that were lying low or that have been niggling us for years, or it strongly exacerbates issues that were previously problems. While this can feel awful, it's great if we can see it as our body signposting what we need to work on.

The gut microbiome was deeply researched for the first time in 2007 with the creation of the Human Microbiome Project, so it's not surprising that we are still learning new insights into this complex part of our body.

There are so many environmental factors that wreak havoc on our gut microbiome. The obvious ones are antibiotics, pesticides, and enzyme inhibitors sprayed on food to keep it looking fresh for longer, but other things such as chemicals in toiletries, common allergens, and refined carbohydrates can be surprisingly damaging.

When we understand how this damage is a major contributor to inflammation in the body and how a compromised immune system is also connected, we stop seeing these issues as interesting facts and they become non-negotiable changes to be made in our lifestyle and diet choices.

As always, let's start at the beginning and explore how the digestive system works.

What is the digestive system?

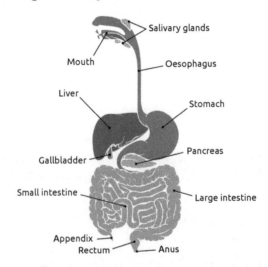

DIAGRAM 13 – THE ANATOMY OF THE DIGESTIVE SYSTEM

The digestive system is a group of organs that work together to turn the food we eat into the energy and nutrients our body needs. These organs are the mouth, oesophagus, stomach, pancreas, small intestine, gallbladder, liver, and large intestine.

When we eat, food travels from the mouth down the oesophagus (throat) to the stomach where it is broken down into its basic parts: carbohydrates, proteins, fats, and nutrients such as vitamins and minerals.

A series of muscle contractions called peristalsis moves the broken-down food through the small and large intestines where the nutrients are absorbed into the bloodstream through the lining of the small intestine. This absorption is controlled by "tight junctions", which are semi-permeable barriers between the cells of the intestine wall.

The leftover broken-down food is compacted until eventually it passes out through the anus as waste.

The liver, pancreas, and gallbladder have important roles as they produce chemicals that allow digestion to occur.

Everything in your body, from your hormones to your heart, requires the nutrients extracted during the digestive process to work correctly.

Digestive issues

However, women commonly experience issues with digestion, not just at menopause but throughout their lives. Issues such as irritable bowel syndrome, gallstones, constipation, or loose stools are more commonly experienced by women than men, which suggests rather strongly that there is a hormonal involvement and a red flag that something isn't right. As with many minor symptoms, these are usually ignored and normalized. If or when the symptoms escalate and become persistent, they will often be medicated to suppress the issue if and where possible, but that doesn't correct the underlying problem.

Let's look at the different organs and the issues that are commonly experienced with them.

The stomach

Millions of menopausal women (and millions of other people) are commonly put on antacids or proton-pump inhibitors, such as omeprazole, due to indigestion, heartburn, and acid reflux.

The stomach is meant to be acidic. If you think back to what happens if we are stressed and sympathetic nervous system dominant, we are not producing the right digestive acid to digest our food. The fact that the use of antacids by menopausal women is so common must stop being normalized. It is true we produce fewer digestive juices as we age, but this would be proportional to a drop in appetite that also happens as we age. If it is not in proportion to appetite, we must be looking at underlying causes of digestive issues and exploring how and why a woman's digestion is under duress. Is it a poor diet? Too much caffeine? Too much stress? Consuming foods she is intolerant to? The stomach is the first major part of our digestion, and medications that inhibit our digestive acid will cause issues further down the road. Problems such as stomach infections (e.g. *Helicobacter pylori*), stomach ulcers, nausea, a worsening of reflux symptoms, postnasal drip, allergies, and inflammatory responses can start here.

Because these medications are considered commonplace, they do not spark the suspicion that they warrant. Although they are meant to be used for short amounts of time, we have seen numerous women be prescribed these for decades. If we cannot digest our food properly, we cannot have hormone health. If we have an issue with digesting our food and experience symptoms, we need to look deeper.

The pancreas

We have talked about the pancreas in depth with regard to blood sugar regulation, and we have previously stated that 95 per cent of its job should be digestion. During digestion, it helps us to break down our food, particularly our fats, so that we can get important nutrients such as vitamin D from them. However, when the pancreas is too busy working on blood sugar regulation, our digestion can be compromised. This issue becomes more obvious in later life for women, with osteoporosis becoming a major concern. It is common to hear of older women fracturing their pelvis or hips after a fall, and these fractures can be due to a lack of vitamin D and undiagnosed insulin resistance.

It is therefore essential that we have a pancreas that can focus on digestion and not just blood sugar stabilization, and it is important to have awareness of the connection between blood sugars, digestion, and osteoporosis, given that menopause is the time that women become aware of the risk of osteoporosis.

The gallbladder

The gallbladder is an interesting organ. It is often disregarded; according to the NHS website, it is not needed and is "removable". Gallstones are commonly experienced by women during their fertile years and in early perimenopause. This is because oestrogen dominance increases cholesterol production, which in turn creates gallstones. However, research also shows that gallstones are connected to insulin resistance as well as gluten, which correlates with our clinical experience of seeing the diets of women who have had gallstones.

The gallbladder stores bile which helps break down fat from food in your intestine. Bile is important: it is antibacterial, supports the health of the microbiome, and regulates the migrating motor complex (MMC), a series of waves that help move food through your digestive system.

The hormone CCK (remember this hormone from Chapter 4?) stimulates the gallbladder to deliver bile into the small intestine, allowing fat-soluble vitamins and nutrients to be more easily absorbed into the bloodstream. Imbalanced blood sugars therefore have a direct impact on our ability to digest food.

Without a gallbladder, we will struggle to break down fats, and, as we know, fats are essential for good hormone health. Women following a low-fat diet as recommended post-surgery for gallbladder removal are going to struggle with hormone production, which may become a problem during the menopause transition.

The liver

Our liver has a big part to play in our health. It performs more than 300 functions and is one the largest and most important organs in the body. Its many functions include:

- production of certain proteins for blood plasma

- production of cholesterol and special proteins to help carry fats through the body

- conversion of excess glucose into glycogen for storage (this glycogen can later be converted back to glucose for energy)

- regulation of blood levels of amino acids, which form the building blocks of proteins

- processing of haemoglobin for use of its iron content

- iron storage

- clearing the blood of drugs and other poisonous substances

- regulating blood clotting

- resisting infections by producing immune factors and removing bacteria from the bloodstream.

But the role we are particularly interested in when it comes to menopause and digestion is what the liver does with detoxing the body.

Detoxing is really misunderstood in the confusing and quickly changing world of nutritional science. Our body detoxes, day in, day out. Fact.

What we tend to mean by "detoxing" is giving our liver a break from the processed foods, caffeine, sugar, and alcohol that we bombard it with, so that it can focus on some of the other jobs it has to do for a while.

However, detoxing is completely misunderstood. Many detoxes focus on eliminating everything except fruit and vegetables from the diet. Juicing is commonly used as a way of accelerating a detox. But it doesn't help us to detox – in fact, it actively stops us from detoxing. To understand this more, let's look at what is happening when the liver is detoxing.

The liver has two phases of detoxification.

Phase 1 is where the liver starts to break down toxic substances into inactive substances. These would be substances like:

- alcohol

- drugs (prescription, over-the-counter, and recreational)

- toxic chemicals from paint, solvents, cleaning products, or toiletries

- pollution.

Now the liver must break them down even further so that the body can eliminate them. This happens during phase 2.

The other thing that happens during phase 2 of detoxification is that the liver also breaks down our metabolic waste. This is where excess hormones are broken down and excreted. All that cortisol, oestrogen, and insulin we have been talking about are processed during this phase of detoxification. As we have been exploring in previous chapters, during perimenopause there can be a lot of hormonal excess due to the pressures of our diet, lifestyle, and the perimenopausal transition.

When we are looking at supporting the body with diet, it is essential to understand that the liver cannot undertake an effective phase 2 detoxification process without two important nutrients: sulphur and amino acids. Both are found in meat and fish protein sources, which are usually removed when "detoxing" and are commonly low in the modern diet.

Diet, lifestyle choices (such as a regular intake of alcohol), and the excess hormone load during perimenopause are massive causes of elevated liver enzymes which show a struggling liver. The knock-on effect with our digestion is that the hormones don't get broken down and cleared out effectively but are recirculated and reabsorbed, overloading our body with hormones it can't utilize.

As we have mentioned previously, another job the liver performs is the manufacture of cholesterol. Elevated cholesterol levels are common during menopause. With regard to digestion, cholesterol is involved in the metabolism of all the fat-soluble vitamins such as vitamin A, D, E, and K. When we consider antioxidants, we think of colourful berries and green leafy vegetables, but cholesterol also acts as an antioxidant.

LDL and HDL

Cholesterol does not dissolve in water, so it cannot travel through your blood on its own. To help transport cholesterol, your liver produces lipoproteins. These lipoproteins are particles made from fat and protein. They carry cholesterol and triglycerides (another type of lipid) through your bloodstream.

The two major forms of lipoprotein are:

- LDL – low-density lipoprotein, commonly known as the "bad cholesterol". LDL picks up cholesterol from the liver and delivers it to cells.

- HDL – high-density lipoprotein, also known as the "good cholesterol". HDL removes excess cholesterol from the blood and takes it to the liver.

It is important to note here that LDL is not "bad". In fact, far from it. Among other things, we need LDL to make our hormones. LDL is also involved in the immune response, acting as a sponge to pick up bacterial toxins.

Those with high cholesterol tend to have one or more of the following factors:

- are overweight or obese

- have insulin resistance

- eat an unhealthy diet full of processed foods and trans fats or a diet high in carbohydrate and low in protein and fat

- do not exercise regularly

- have a high-stress lifestyle

- smoke

- have a family history of high cholesterol

- have diabetes, kidney disease, or hypothyroidism

- have an underlying issue with the gut microbiome.

Elevated levels of cholesterol are a symptom of the underlying problem, not the cause of the problem. The underlying issue is inflammation caused by the factors mentioned in the list above.

When our body becomes inflamed, the blood vessels and arteries literally swell up and develop microscopic tears in their walls. A tear in an artery wall can be fatal, so before it becomes a major issue, cholesterol is sent as a rescuer to the artery to heal the inflammation. If it is successful, everything returns to normal.

If the inflammation does not subside, more cholesterol is sent and starts to accumulate around the artery as a band-aid. This is how plaque starts to form. Cholesterol is the firefighter being blamed for the fire.

Pretty much everything we have talked about in every chapter so far is to do with the causes of inflammation:

- imbalanced blood sugars

- high stress

- gut dysbiosis

- environmental toxins

- medications including the pill and synthetic HRT

- infections

- smoking and drinking alcohol

- autoimmune conditions (those with autoimmune disorders tend to have higher cholesterol).

Cholesterol reduction

The traditional advice for improving cholesterol includes avoiding saturated fats, limiting cholesterol in food, cutting back on eggs or eating only egg whites, limiting red meat, and drinking low-fat milk.

This is a very reductionist view because saturated fats provide cell membrane integrity and enhance the body's ability to use essential fatty acids. They protect the liver and are the preferred food for the heart and brain. Dietary cholesterol contributes to the strength of the intestinal wall and helps babies and children develop a healthy brain and nervous system. Foods that contain cholesterol also contain other nutrients. Grass-fed red meat and eggs are a rich source of nutrients, and processed milks and low-fat and non-fat milk lack fat-soluble vitamins needed to assimilate the protein and minerals in the milk itself, which in turn causes more inflammation.

Statins are also commonly recommended. They work to decrease cholesterol levels in your body. They do this by blocking the body's production of an enzyme called HMG-CoA reductase. This is the enzyme your liver needs to make cholesterol. Blocking this enzyme causes your liver to make less cholesterol, which in turn lowers your cholesterol levels. Statins also work by making it easier for the body to absorb cholesterol that is already built up in the arteries. Statins might deal with the symptom, but they do not address the underlying problem and, in fact, can contribute to the problem as they

— 104 —

also increase insulin resistance and insulin secretion, which is a major cause of inflammation.

To reduce cholesterol, we need to go back to the Triangle of Hormonal Health – balancing the blood sugars, reducing stress, finding the right way to balance our hormones during the menopause transition, and reducing dysbiosis in the gut.

Which leads us on to...

The small intestine

The small intestine (or small bowel) is much longer than the large intestine, but it's called the small intestine because it is narrower. It is here that we absorb all the nutrients from our broken-down food, but it is also where we can experience a lot of digestive issues.

In fact, a lot of our time as coaches is spent trying to support people to understand what is going on in their small intestine and what to do about it.

Common issues associated with the small intestine that women tend to be dealing with, not only during menopause but often for decades prior to menopause, are irritable bowel syndrome and small intestine bacterial overgrowth (SIBO).

Irritable bowel syndrome

Irritable bowel syndrome is a common condition that causes symptoms such as cramps, bloating, diarrhoea, constipation, and nausea. These symptoms tend to come and go and are usually triggered by food or emotional experiences. It is considered a functional disorder as it generally doesn't progress to become a disease of the bowel such as Crohn's disease.

It is, however, a hideous and, in some cases, life-affecting condition. We both know the IBS story too well, having both suffered terribly since our teens. In fact, it was trying to find a solution to IBS that led to the creation of our first protocol and kick-started our research into hormones. The "aha" moment came when a gastroenterologist friend of ours once said, "The IBS will go away when you hit menopause and your hormones change." When we asked why, he said it's all to do with "oestrogen, stress, and food intolerance". When we asked why endocrinologists don't deal with it if it is rooted in hormonal disturbance, the answer was simply that because it shows up in the gut, it is dealt with by gut doctors, not hormone doctors.

In the medical model, there is currently no known cause of IBS and no known cure. The low-FODMAP diet is often used, but success is low (only around 20% of people find an improvement). In some cases antidepressants are offered to reduce symptoms, but, again, the results are hit and miss.

However, in recent years some interesting connections have been made between IBS and SIBO.

But before we dive into that juicy topic, we want to talk about an important structure in the bowel. Many complementary therapies tout an imbalance in this structure as the "cause" of IBS; however, we see it as a victim of what is going on in the bowel, not the main issue.

The ileocecal valve (ICV)

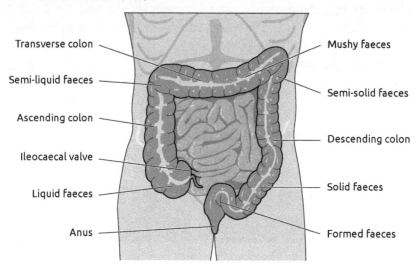

DIAGRAM 14 – THE POSITION OF THE ILEOCECAL VALVE

Located between the small intestine and the large intestine is a valve called the ileocecal valve (ICV). The purpose of this valve is to "prevent backflow" from the large intestine, where we turn broken-down food into poo, back into the small intestine, where we absorb nutrients from the broken-down food (called chyme).

The chyme approaches the ICV and the ICV opens. Once the food passes through, the ICV shuts again.

The appendix sits behind the ileocecal valve in the large intestine. This is also a misunderstood and highly useful structure, whose job it is to squirt the chyme that has passed through the ICV and entered the large intestine with a mucus that has bacteria designed to keep our intestines healthy and an enzyme that breaks down plant food.

In therapies like kinesiology and chiropractic, it is taught that a malfunctioning ileocecal valve is behind a lot of common symptoms.

What we mean by malfunctioning is that it will either get stuck shut, stopping food from passing through to the large intestine, or get stuck open, meaning that faecal matter can leak back to the small intestine where it can be reabsorbed, which can contribute to a lot of symptoms such as:

- joint pain
- muscular aches and pains
- shoulder or neck pain
- sudden, stabbing, sharp low-back pain
- dull headaches
- migraines
- chronic sinus infection, dripping sinuses
- allergies
- dark circles under the eyes, puffy cheeks
- constipation
- loose bowels or diarrhoea
- asthma-like symptoms
- general non-specific lower gastrointestinal discomfort
- bloating.

The ICV malfunctions for a variety of reasons, including a high-carbohydrate/low-protein diet or a diet high in processed food, emotional stress, postural misalignment (especially from hip issues), jaw problems, and upper-thigh or gluteus muscle wastage, SIBO, food intolerance, and dehydration.

There is, however, a major hormonal connection here, and it was our research into this area that led to the creation of our theory called…

The bowel hormone storm

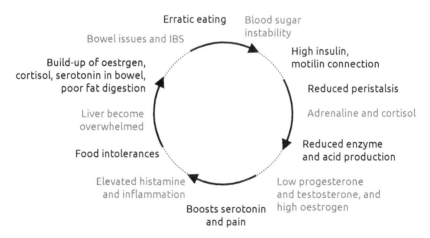

DIAGRAM 15 – HOW HORMONES AFFECT BOWEL FUNCTION

And it goes something like this…

When we eat a diet that is high in carbohydrate, highly processed, or containing inflammatory foods or foods we are intolerant to, we imbalance our blood sugars.

This has a knock-on effect, with digestive hormones such as motilin, a hormone that stimulates small intestine motility, causing undigested food to move into the large intestine.

Imbalanced blood sugars cause adrenaline and cortisol to spike, which increases the acid in the stomach and reduces enzyme output from the pancreas. This also slows down peristalsis, causing the griping sensations we know too well if we have experienced gut problems.

With heightened stress, we see the leg muscles rotate, which can misalign the pelvis. This in turn misaligns the ICV, which causes digestive disturbance and pain.

With high insulin, high cortisol, and impaired motilin and serotonin, we see an increase in stress and oestrogen and a reduction in the production of progesterone.

High oestrogen and gut disturbance contribute to high histamine, increased inflammation, and a heightened immune response, which can show itself as allergies or food intolerances.

If the body is unable to process and balance these hormones, we stay in the blood sugar rollercoaster which adds to our desire to eat erratically.

And around and around we go...

While this is happening, we are in a situation of creating an adverse environment in our gut microbiome, which then contributes to a change in the gut flora and a predisposition to developing issues like SIBO. This becomes more common during perimenopause as we are naturally battling the issue of increased insulin resistance and the reduction in progesterone.

On top of this, once we have repeated inflammation in the gut, we are increasing the chances of "intestinal permeability" (often called "leaky gut"), which is when the tight junctions develop impairments and allow substances through the gut wall and into the bloodstream. Intestinal permeability is behind so many conditions including arthritis, brain fog, autoimmune diseases, and certain cancers.

The gut-associated lymphoid tissues (GALT) in the small intestine house approximately 80 percent of the body's immune system and can be considered the root cause of chronic inflammatory diseases (more on this in the next chapter), but part of this is that if we have inflammation here as well as elevated oestrogen, we will have an increase in histamine, which accounts for why so many women suddenly become intolerant to seemingly random foods during menopause.

We've already mentioned it a few times now, but let's cut to the chase and talk about SIBO.

What is SIBO?

Normally, very few bacteria should be able to survive in the upper small intestine. However, huge numbers of bacteria live in the lower part of the small intestine. They have a very important role here, helping with the digestion of food.

When the environment or the function of the small intestine is adversely affected, as illustrated by the bowel hormone storm, bacteria can multiply and live within some or all of the small intestines. This is called "small intestinal bacterial overgrowth". Bacteria are classified as either gram-negative or gram-positive based on the structure of their cell wall. Many common pathogens are gram-negative, such as *E. coli* and *Salmonella*. SIBO tend to also be gram-negative.

Gram-negative bacteria have a thin, hard-to-penetrate cell membrane, which is resistant to many antibiotics like penicillin and means that they can be challenging to get under control.

One of the major issues with SIBO is that they have a substance present in their membrane called an endotoxin. These endotoxins are chemicals called lipopolysaccharides.

Endotoxins are an extremely strong stimulator of the immune system. At low levels, endotoxins cause chronic systemic inflammation and are linked to intestinal permeability, obesity, diabetes, cardiovascular disease, and autoimmune disease; at high levels, endotoxins cause septic shock. They also mimic oestrogen as a xeno-oestrogen.

What else causes SIBO?

Perimenopause is the perfect storm for SIBO developing: the insulin resistance, high cortisol, high oestrogen, and low progesterone are exactly the environment for SIBO.

A common cycle we see in perimenopause, due to dropping and fluctuating sex hormones, is that women can experience reoccurring infections such as UTIs (urinary tract infections). The medical answer is antibiotics, and therefore women can find themselves on repeated courses of antibiotics which disrupt the gut environment; in turn, this triggers an immune response and creates further infections. And round and round we go.

Combine that with a poor diet, and it's no surprise we see so much of it. However, there are also other causes, including:

- thyroid conditions

- low levels of stomach acid

- acid reflux or gastroesophageal reflux disease (GERD)

- medications such as omeprazole or overuse of antacids such as Gaviscon
- physical abnormalities of the small intestine
- a weakened immune system
- antibiotic usage
- the pill
- food poisoning
- gut infections
- frequent sugar, carbohydrate, or alcohol consumption.

When the bacteria in the upper small bowel reach high enough numbers, they start to cause symptoms. These can include:

- stomach or abdominal pain
- belching
- IBS (studies showed a high number of people with IBS also have SIBO present)
- bloating after eating (exacerbated after taking probiotics or eating fermented foods)
- diarrhoea
- constipation
- ileocecal valve pain
- nausea
- unintentional weight loss
- malabsorption of key nutrients including B12, iron, and the fat-soluble vitamins including A, D, E, and K – this is because their hard-to-penetrate cell membranes mean that they create a lining in the small intestine so we can't absorb nutrients
- autoimmune conditions – due to the connection with intestinal permeability
- inflammation – due to the connection with endotoxins and intestinal permeability

DIGESTIVE FUNCTION

- food intolerances

- high histamine – the body produces enzymes in the digestive tract (diamine oxidase – DAO) to keep histamine in check; SIBO inhibits the body from producing this enzyme and causes histamine to build up; this is why clients with SIBO often have allergies and regular histamine response

- production of the bacteria *Lactobacillus casei* and *L. bulgaricus*, which stimulate the production of histamine

- fats in stools (the bacteria metabolize bile salts making it difficult to process fats)

- skin issues such as rosacea, psoriasis, rashes, and eczema

- nausea

- joint pain

- fatigue

- sleep issues

- gallbladder issues including stones.

Another interesting correlation to note is that research shows people with higher levels of endotoxins experience depression, suicidal thoughts, apathy, and confusion; these symptoms are commonly attributed to another cause and, even in some cases, medicated.

How do we get rid of it?

It's a good question. SIBO can be stubborn, and it can come back time and time again. Many medical doctors don't recognize SIBO. Those who do diagnose it using a breath test that identifies excess methane or hydrogen in the gut after exposure to carbohydrates.

If the test is positive, they will offer targeted antibiotics, but the results can be hit and miss, as it is essential to get the environment rebalanced prior to treatment with antibiotics and then reinoculated with probiotics (if they can be tolerated).

Diet is an incredibly effective tool to deal with SIBO. We talk about diet in Part Two, but the research into a keto-carnivore diet in relation to SIBO is fascinating stuff.

If a full elimination diet sounds too extreme, a gentler approach using herbs such as oregano oil can be very helpful but just take a bit longer.

Large intestine

Finally, our digestion journey ends with the large intestine.

The large intestine is where we compact the chyme and turn it into faeces, and where we absorb water and iron. Common problems with the large intestine are constipation and diarrhoea, but these are usually more to do with diet or issues further up the digestive tract. Conditions such as diverticulitis, where the intestine distorts to create pouches, can again be linked to diet and problems further up the digestive tract.

The large intestine contains many of the bacteria in the gut microbiome. There are 1000 times more bacteria per gram compared to the ileum and 10,000,000 times more compared to the stomach and duodenum.

What is the gut microbiome?

There are microbiomes in different places including our eyes, skin, vagina, and mouth, but the most important, and the most damaged by our current lifestyles, is the gut microbiome. Our gut microbiome is made up of billions of bacteria, viruses, fungi, and parasites that work together as an amazing colony and literally define how healthy we are.

Not only does the gut microbiome have a huge part to play in digestion, but it also constitutes the largest part of our immune system.

But it's struggling with our modern lifestyle.

The bacteria are incredibly sensitive. If we go back to the environmental factors affecting our health, we must look at pesticides on our food and our exposure to pollution. The problem is that these chemicals disrupt the natural behaviour of bacteria and fungi and kill them off. This is great when that "pest" is causing your potatoes to become plagued with blight, but not great when they are bacteria in your body trying to fight off infections and disease.

Now add in antibiotics and medications that can cause bacteria disruption (by the very definition of antibiotics), and we have a situation that is killing off our gut microbiome, that reduces our ability to digest and metabolize, and that reduces our immunity and causes even more inflammation.

Part of this amazing system is something called the oestrobolome.

After our liver has broken down oestrogen, as discussed previously, it sends it off to the intestines for elimination as waste or reabsorption. In the case of reabsorption, it means that the oestrogen will be recirculated throughout our body. This process is guided by gut bacteria which produce an enzyme called beta-glucuronidase, which in turn breaks down the oestrogen.

This process means we can make oestrogen in a form our body can use from the naturally occurring compounds in plants called phyto-oestrogens, such as soya.

A healthy oestrobolome should block oestrogen receptors when levels are too high and make more when oestrogen levels are low, but this will only work if our gut microbiome is healthy.

Xeno-oestrogens from chemicals, pesticides, and pollution are part of the reason the oestrobolome becomes imbalanced and why it damages our gut microbiome.

Endometriosis and the gut

Many women are entering perimenopause with a history of endometriosis.

Recent studies indicate that gut microbial diversity is altered and significantly lower in patients with endometriosis.[1] It is believed that the gut microbiome is involved because of the inflammatory response caused by a damaged microbiome, intestinal permeability, and the knock-on effect of oestrogen metabolism. As a result, women with a history of endometriosis and of using contraceptives to try to keep the condition under control could struggle during perimenopause when trying to balance their hormones. The use of natural progesterone as HRT has been shown to be helpful for endometriosis.

But our digestive organs and microbiome aren't the only pieces of the puzzle when it comes to good gut health. Another very important and over-looked piece is the vagus nerve. This is another aspect where we start to see all the aspects of the triangle start to come together.

The vagus nerve and gut health

The word "vagus" means wandering in Latin. This is a very appropriate name, as the vagus nerve is the longest cranial nerve. It runs all the way from the brain stem to the colon. It stops just before the descending colon in the large intestine.

Researchers have discovered a connection between high vagal tone and positive emotions and physical health. It is also part of the system that helps us to feel safe in the world. According to the "polyvagal theory", many of our historic reactions and responses to danger and shock can be stored in the vagus nerve.[2]

The vagus nerve is closely associated with four other nerves, and this group are involved in chewing, swallowing, and facial expressions.

Good vagal tone is important in ensuring we go into the parasympathetic nervous system response which allows us to wind down, relax, and digest our food.

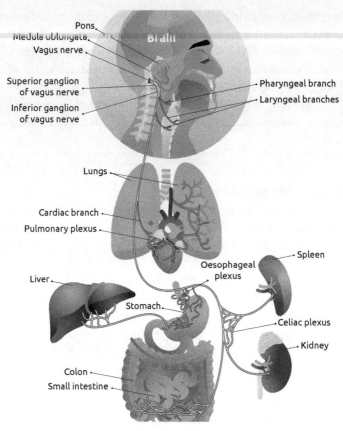

DIAGRAM 16 – THE ANATOMY OF THE VAGUS NERVE

Role of the vagus nerve

- Helps the body relax
- Direct communication between the gut and the brain
- Swallowing
- Increases gastric juices
- Calms fight-or-flight response
- Reduces inflammation and calms the immune response
- Helps with breathing
- Helps with memory
- Controls heart rate

Symptoms of vagus nerve dysfunction

- Fainting
- Chronic inflammation
- Inflammatory disorders such as IBD or colitis

- Digestive issues
- Socialization problems
- Hoarse, croaky, wheezy voice
- Trouble drinking liquids
- Gag reflex difficulty
- Ear pain
- Unusual heart rate
- Abnormal blood pressure
- Nausea or vomiting
- Decreased production of stomach acid
- Abdominal bloating or pain
- Fluctuations in blood sugar

As you can see, the vagus nerve can be part of all sides of the triangle that we have previously discussed.

What is fascinating is how much it is connected to our gut. The vagus nerve is one of the key players in modulating the permeability of our intestinal barrier, so it has a huge part to play in determining whether we develop intestinal permeability. The vagus nerve signifies to our gut that we are stressed, which increases the permeability. But the vagus nerve is also activated by the gut microbiome as the microbiota transmits information to the brain via the vagus nerve. This is how the gut–brain axis works. The gut will be sending data to your brain, which helps your brain determine mood, pain levels, stress, and hunger.

The Triangle of Hormonal Health and how it affects digestive function

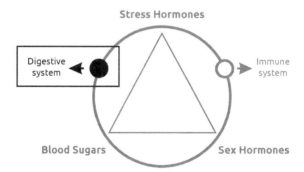

DIAGRAM 17 – THE TRIANGLE OF HORMONAL HEALTH FOCUSING ON DIGESTIVE FUNCTION

This is where the Triangle of Hormonal Health comes into its own. Digestive issues are commonly looked at very myopically by both the medical model and the complementary health world. But this is where we miss key information because issues in our digestive system are usually rooted in one or more of the hormone systems in the triangle.

Blood sugars

Imbalanced blood sugars are hugely implicated in digestive issues. Unstable blood sugars contribute to lack of gut motility, bloating, digestive pain, and an inability to break down fats.

Stress hormones

Stress hormones are connected because of the correlation with the ICV and the reduction in creation of digestive enzymes, and the vagus nerve communication with the gut and the parasympathetic nervous system.

Sex hormones

Sex hormones are involved because too little progesterone will increase the levels of cortisol, and too much oestrogen will cause issues in the oestrobolome. High or low oestrogen and progesterone levels can cause digestive issues like diarrhoea, stomach pain, bloating, and nausea.

Immune function

Gut dysbiosis and intestinal permeability are major causes of inflammation and affect our whole immune response.

It's essential, then, to get the foundations right in terms of diet, reducing stress, and doing what we can to balance hormone confusion, such as the presence of xeno-oestrogens, in order to have a healthy gut and digestive system.

TAKE-HOME MESSAGE

Our gut is hugely involved not only in how we digest our food but also in how we metabolize hormones and in determining our mood, our hunger, our stress levels, and our overall wellbeing. Having a healthy gut microbiome is essential, and microbiome issues such as SIBO can have a huge knock-on effect. Ultimately, much of this can be supported by restabilizing our Triangle of Hormonal Health and restoring balance to our hormones! HRT won't work effectively if we don't have a healthy gut!

— CHAPTER 8 —

Immune function

The immune system and hormones are inextricably linked, and when viewed through the lens of the triangle, we can see the immune system is a victim of instability in the Triangle of Hormonal Health.

Viewing the immune system this way becomes compelling. Research shows the significant disparity between sexes when it comes to autoimmune disease. A staggering 80 per cent of diagnosed autoimmune patients are female. Furthermore, there are strong links suggesting that diverging sex hormone levels during the reproductive years are implicated in autoimmune disease development.[1]

Testosterone, which is more dominant in men, is shown to be anti-inflammatory and immune protective, whereas oestrogen is both pro-inflammatory and has anti-inflammatory roles depending on the job it is doing and whether we have the right amount of it.

Oestrogen plays a complex role in the hormonal response to inflammation. It can be anti-inflammatory (e.g. during pregnancy) but also pro-inflammatory (e.g. in autoimmune diseases) depending on the combination of challenges the immune and systemic response systems are dealing with.[2]

Women can experience immune system issues throughout their whole life, not just during the menopause, but periods of hormonal change such as pregnancy and the menopause either shine a light on issues and bring them to the fore or send them into remission.

Sadly, the medical approach to many conditions, including allergies, intolerances, repeated colds or infections, and systemic inflammation, is to give medication such as anti-inflammatories, antibiotics, antihistamines, or even steroids, rather than taking a wider look at the health history of the woman in front of them, which often shows a picture of hormone destabilization. This approach therefore doesn't take into consideration that natural body-identical HRT (which we will explore in Part Two) has an anti-inflammatory, immune-supporting action.

Let's have a look at what the immune system is and how it works.

The immune system is a highly complex, integrated collection of organs, cells, and chemicals that protects the body internally and externally from threats, injury, and disease. It defends us from pathogens (viruses, bacteria, parasites, fungi), removes foreign objects, heals wounds, repairs and maintains tissue, and detects and eliminates cancer cells. However, when the immune system goes awry and doesn't function correctly, we see issues such as systemic inflammation, chronic allergies, infections, autoimmune disease, or cancer. It is easy to consider that the immune system is broken, but we believe it is more useful to take the view that an imbalanced immune system is highlighting that there is an issue with the internal or external environment of the body. The common misconception with the immune system is that this system is only focused on trying to deal with pathogens coming to "get us", when it is the state of our internal environment that governs whether we can deal with pathogens.

There are hundreds of cells and functions involved in this intricate system, but to start to understand how it works, we just need some basic information.

In the immune system, we have T cells and B cells. These are the soldiers of the immune system army, and they are mostly made in our bone marrow.

T cells are responsible for dealing with pathogens and invaders that occur inside our cells.

B cells are responsible for dealing with pathogens and invaders that occur outside of our cells.

We then have structures and other systems that are involved in transmitting information about what is needed from T and B cells.

Tonsils and adenoids: These an early warning system detecting pathogens and food allergens. Imagine these as the warning lights on your dashboard. These two organs are commonly removed because they are seen as not having an important function; however, both play a role in immune system communication and protection.

Thymus gland: As we know from Chapter 5 on stress, the thymus is part of the endocrine system. It produces the hormone thymosin which helps to make T cells. The thymus is where our T cells mature and learn to differentiate between our own cells and foreign invaders. Think of the thymus as a school for T cells.

Spleen: Our spleen stores red blood cells and T and B cells, and filters blood, removing old blood cells and making sure only undamaged effective cells are left.

Liver: A surprising one, but the liver can be considered an organ of the immune system. The liver houses cells that engulf and absorb bacteria, produces natural killer cells which remove cells that are tumorous or have been infected by a virus, as well as manufacturing antigen-presenting cells, which basically means presenting information to T cells to do their job. The liver is needed to work so hard at times of metabolic distress that it really is essential to look after it and make sure that it isn't working too hard, so that when we need it to do its job, it can. Constantly bombarding it with processed food, alcohol, and toxins means it can't step up when we need it to.

Lymphatic vessels and nodes: These are the filter stations containing different immune cells that trap pathogens and activate antibodies.

Skin and mucous membranes: Your skin is the first line of defence in preventing and destroying germs before they enter your body. Skin produces oils and secretes other protective immune system cells. Mucous membranes line the respiratory, digestive, urinary, and reproductive tracts. Mucus is needed to lubricate and moisten surfaces. Germs stick to mucus in the respiratory tract and then are moved out of the airways. Tiny hairs in your nose catch germs. Enzymes found in sweat, tears, saliva, and mucous membranes as well as secretions in the vagina all defend against and destroy germs.

We also know from the previous chapter that our gut is hugely involved in our immune system. Specifically, this includes our appendix, which is part of the GALT, our stomach and bowel because of the regulation of acid to help in killing off unwanted bacteria, and Peyer's patches, which are in mucosa of the small intestine and monitor intestinal bacteria to keep it maintained.

As well as T and B cells, and structures and organs, we also have T-helper cells or TH cells. These are the commanders of our immune system army, sending signals to guide the T and B cells to attack or stand down.

There are many types of TH cells but the ones that are important for our purposes are:

- **TH1 cells,** which instruct T cells. This is our immediate response to attackers *inside* the cell – our first line of defence. The response is to create inflammation.

- **TH2 cells,** which instruct B cells. TH2 cells aim to destroy pathogens such as viruses, bacteria, toxins, and allergens that occur *outside* our cells. This is a slower response, and it is anti-inflammatory.

In a well-functioning immune system, TH1 and TH2 cells work together to keep the system in balance. When a threat is recognized by the immune system, first the TH1 cells are sent; after the invader has been dealt with,

IMPROVING THE MENOPAUSE EXPERIENCE THROUGH NUTRITION AND LIFESTYLE

TH2 cells are deployed. One side might become more active to eradicate a threat, and the body goes back to balance. However, with cancer, TH2 cells can be elevated, and with autoimmune conditions, TH1 cells can be elevated.

The reason all of this is important during the menopause transition is because oestrogen and progesterone have a powerful effect on the immune system. As both hormones decline during menopause, we see a drop in our immune response or an increase in conditions such as autoimmune disease. This is because the depletion of progesterone and oestrogen results in a drop in the concentration of T cells. Conversely, if oestrogen is too high (or progesterone is low), it will affect our immune response because of the inflammatory nature of being oestrogen dominant.

What is inflammation?

We've talked a lot about inflammation, but what is it?

Basically, it is the immune system responding to an irritant. That irritant can be coming from inside the body or outside the body. However, there are two types of inflammation.

Acute inflammation is an injury or infection that clears up within days or weeks. If you bang your knee, for example, the swelling, bruising, pain, and heat are all part of the acute inflammatory response and the body repairing the damage that's happened. The word "inflammation" comes from the Latin *inflammare*, meaning "to set on fire", and even though it's horrible to experience, it's an important and necessary process of your body healing.

In acute inflammation, the first line of defence comes from a part of the immune system called the innate immune system. This part of the system is activated quickly. Once the innate immune system has been sent to the scene and has started to address the issue, the adaptive immune system is called in. The adaptive immune system is more intelligent and has more sophisticated tools than the innate system, and it can learn from the situation to better prepare the body for future scenarios.

Chronic inflammation is different from banging your knee or getting a cold. It is the slow, long-term type of inflammation that lasts for several months or years and is a driver of chronic health conditions such as auto-immune diseases and type 2 diabetes. Chronic inflammation is damage that the body's immune system is trying to repair but can't. This can be because the damage is ongoing and continuous such as exposure to toxic chemicals in our environment, gut damage from repeatedly eating poor food choices, oestrogen dominance in perimenopause, or taking certain medications such as the pill. Chronic inflammation uses a different mechanism compared to acute inflammation. It's the adaptive immune response that is dealing with

— 120 —

chronic inflammation and it requests excessive and repeated activation of innate immune cells because it can't heal the problem.

Chronic inflammation is a growing issue in our modern lives. The medical approach focuses on reducing chronic inflammation without asking or addressing why it's there. An example of this is prescribing statins, which reduce cholesterol but misunderstand that the cholesterol is there to put out the fire of chronic inflammation caused by our diet and lifestyle.

Menopause and autoimmune disease

There are around 80 autoimmune diseases that range in severity from mild to disabling. Many of these conditions have been normalized, such as a small patch of psoriasis or eczema, or childhood asthma, but we would argue that if the immune system is in an autoimmune response, it is a red flag that needs to be taken seriously.

The medical approach to most autoimmune conditions is that the body is mistakenly attacking itself, and they will prescribe steroids either topically or systemically, which suppress the immune response with high doses of the anti-inflammatory cortisol derivative cortisone.

But when we look at how the human body has evolved, it is unlikely that someone has developed psoriasis or eczema, or multiple sclerosis, because they are deficient in a high dose of cortisone or that the body is mistaken. Again, we need to go back to inflammation, and for that we need to return to the gut.

As we have discussed in Chapter 7 on the digestive function, menopausal women are predisposed to increased bacterial growth in the gut because of the decrease in sex hormones. This can result in the development of SIBO, food intolerances, allergies, and other intestinal symptoms.

For many years, the naturopathic industry has been talking about a poor gut environment and leaky gut (or intestinal permeability) being at the core of immune conditions. This is a challenge menopausal women face because they are naturally in a state of hormone imbalance, which increases the risk of intestinal permeability.

As we've previously explored, only relatively small molecules should cross the gut barrier to enter the body, but when intestinal permeability is present, microscopic holes are formed through which some of the contents of the gut can leak into the bloodstream or lymphatic system. The molecules that are meant to stay in the gut – pathogens, incompletely digested proteins, bacteria, infectious organisms, toxic substances, or waste products that would normally be excreted – can "leak" into the bloodstream.

This triggers the immune system because it recognizes these particles as foreign invaders and mounts a response against them. When this happens with regularity, the liver sees that there is body-wide inflammation, and this sends the immune system into overdrive.

This interplay is at the heart of autoimmune disorders and why peri-menopausal women are more at risk of an autoimmune diagnosis. For this situation to become an autoimmune response, a specific TH cell called TH17 creates "autoantibodies" where the antibody attacks body tissue instead of a pathogen.

However, some very progressive doctors are now also linking this intestinal permeability and the systemic inflammation it can cause to certain cancers.

Menopause and cancer

Cancer is increasing dramatically, with one in two people receiving a diagnosis at some point during their lifetime.

Breast cancer is the most common type of cancer in the UK, and most women who are diagnosed are over the age of 50 and going through the menopause transition.

Since the 1950s, breast cancer occurrence has risen by 60 per cent, and it would therefore appear that there is something about our modern life that is carcinogenic.

This is a sensitive subject to discuss. As complementary health practitioners and nutritionists, we cannot diagnose, treat, or work with cancer, but with so many new cases being diagnosed, especially during menopause, it is an important issue to explore.

Cancer is misunderstood, and advertising for cancer charities tends to focus on the enemy within that is trying to attack and kill us. This is not the case. All cancers start with a minor change within a cell, and this is a sign that there is an imbalance in the body.

Although we are at higher risk if someone in our family has had cancer, there are many lifestyle factors that are also strong drivers for cancer developing, including:

- **physical** carcinogens, such as radiation

- **chemical** carcinogens, such as tobacco smoke, alcohol, and drinking water contaminants

- **biological** carcinogens, such as hormone imbalance, infections from certain viruses, bacteria, or parasites and intestinal permeability.

Hormonally induced cancers – namely, breast, endometrial, ovarian, and thyroid cancer and osteosarcoma – often occur due to an imbalance of oestrogen and progesterone.

However, the only known cause of endometrial cancer is unopposed oestrogens, meaning too much oestrogen being present without progesterone to balance it out. Breast cancer is also more likely to occur in premenopausal women with normal or high oestrogen levels and low progesterone. Women using the combined pill, which contains high levels of oestrogen, have been shown to have three times the risk of developing cancer compared to non-pill users.

Although cancer and autoimmune disease appear to be different, they can be seen as two sides of the same coin. Autoimmune disease results from an elevated immune response, while cancer develops when the immune system does not respond to malignant cells. One condition is an overreactive immune response, and the other is an underactive immune response.

The moral of this story is that if we enter perimenopause with high stress, poor diet, using medications that are affecting our hormones, high alcohol, drug, or nicotine use, and exposure to hormone-disrupting chemicals, our detoxification organs such as the lungs, kidneys, and bowel can be compromised and unable to deal with the added stress of menopause. There is then a greater risk of conditions such as autoimmune disease or cancer.

However, there are other signs of dysfunction in the immune system – it's not just the big things like autoimmune disease and cancer.

Menopause and histamine

During menopause, many women can experience symptoms due to high histamine and histamine intolerance.

Histamine is a hormone mainly known for its role in an allergic response, but histamine has other important functions, including regulating the sleep–wake cycle (the circadian rhythm), improving cognitive function, and regulating stomach acid, ovulation, and libido.

We have histamine receptors throughout most organs and tissues in our body, including the central nervous system and the gastrointestinal tract, which is why histamine can affect the whole body.

It can be difficult to distinguish between high histamine or histamine intolerance and an actual allergy, and it is common for perimenopausal women to suddenly develop intolerances and allergic responses, or insomnia and brain fog, out of the blue, because of the hormonal changes happening. One of the sentences we hear commonly in clinic is "I have always eaten oysters/eggs/mussels/fish/sauerkraut [or insert other foodstuffs here] and then I ate it and suddenly felt headachy/sick/stomach pains."

High histamine symptoms include:

- headaches
- anxiety
- insomnia
- brain fog
- hives, rashes, and skin itching
- nasal congestion
- irritable bowel syndrome
- skin conditions such as eczema.

It is more common in women because oestrogen stimulates a special type of white blood cell called mast cells to make more histamine. At the same time, oestrogen suppresses an enzyme called diamine oxidase (DAO) which clears histamine. Histamine then stimulates the ovaries to make more oestrogen, so the oestrogen/histamine relationship is a vicious cycle.

More oestrogen → more histamine → more oestrogen → more histamine

As well as histamine made in the body, it is also present in the foods we eat, such as fermented foods, and in our environment. For example, our reaction to stinging nettles is a direct response to the histamine present in the plant. If you are having an immune response to a glass of red wine, it could be the histamine present in the wine.

There are many factors that cause high histamine. Foods such as gluten and dairy stimulate histamine release if we are intolerant to them, and some food such as red wine, sauerkraut, and cured meat contain a lot of histamine. The oestrogen dominance that occurs in perimenopause will trigger the histamine/oestrogen cycle, and some medications such as antibiotics and antidepressants stimulate histamine. Histamine is also created in response to other systemic inflammation as part of the immune response.

In a healthy functioning body, we should be able to clear the excess histamine, but commonly in perimenopause this doesn't happen due to a variety of issues such as SIBO, which impairs DAO activity and stops histamine being cleared in the gut, as well as oestrogen dominance and progesterone deficiency, which suppresses DAO. HRT can also create oestrogen excess, which stimulates the creation of histamine. Gut dysbiosis also affects histamine clearing. If we have a lack of vitamin B6 or magnesium, we won't make enough DAO. Basically, everything we are navigating in perimenopause can stimulate the production of histamine and reduce our ability to clear it out.

One of the reasons that histamine issues can be overlooked as part of perimenopause is because our body releases higher levels of histamine naturally at night as well as after meals. When this happens, the body tries to release built-up histamine, and the symptoms of this include flushing, itching, difficulty regulating body temperature, heart palpitations, and sudden excessive sweating, which are almost identical to symptoms of the menopause itself.

Commonly, women are mistakenly given oestrogen HRT as the GP believes their symptoms are being driven by an oestrogen deficiency, but the opposite could be true. High oestrogen is driving the high histamine symptoms. This is why women can feel worse on oestrogen HRT.

The immune toxic overload reaction

Any build-up of toxins in the body causes hormone disruption, immune responses, and inflammation.

From the air we breathe, the food we eat, the water we drink, and the products we put on our bodies and clean our houses with, almost everything contains levels of unwanted substances that our body must metabolize and excrete, so as not to allow build-up which damages our tissues. We are exposed to literally hundreds of toxic chemicals. We are going to explore how to spot them and avoid them in Part Two, but for now it's important to understand how they affect the immune system.

When your body's toxic burden exceeds a healthy threshold, it kicks the immune system into overdrive, leading to increased inflammation and immune dysregulation.

Environmental toxins also shrink the thymus, which is a small organ just behind your lungs where immune cells go to mature. When the thymus shrinks in response to toxin exposure, there's a diminished production of T regulatory cells. All of this contributes to the change in immune function.

The Triangle of Hormonal Health and how it affects immune function

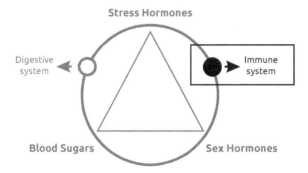

DIAGRAM 18 – THE TRIANGLE OF HORMONAL HEALTH FOCUSING ON THE IMMUNE SYSTEM

The immune system can be seen as the ultimate victim of the Triangle of

Hormonal Health because when the triangle is imbalanced, we see a big knock-on effect with immune function.

Blood sugars

Blood sugar hormones leptin and ghrelin reduce inflammation when in balance, but stimulate inflammation when out of balance.

Insulin stimulates an immune system response.

Stress hormones

When we have blood sugar instability and inflammation, we produce more cortisol, which in turn spikes blood sugars.

Sex hormones

Elevated cortisol reduces our ability to make progesterone, leading to oestrogen dominance, which is immune stimulating.

We are also progesterone deficient naturally at perimenopause, leading to oestrogen dominance, which is an immune stimulant.

Digestive function

Elevated insulin, cortisol, and oestrogen disrupt the gut microbiome and can lead to dysbiosis and intestinal permeability, triggering repeated immune responses.

Oestrogen stimulates mast cells to make more histamine, elevating the immune response.

Events that trigger chronic conditions

When we are in this place of an unstable Triangle of Hormonal Health, we are susceptible to chronic conditions. Many of the women we work with have a history of fatigue disorders and autoimmune conditions.

We hope you can see, from all that we have illustrated previously, that these don't come out of the blue. Commonly, a major chronic condition has a trigger event, which people think is when the issue started. The truth is that the scene was set years before.

When you have a body with an imbalanced Triangle of Hormonal Health, including poor diet, high stress, imbalanced hormones, unhealthy gut environment, and a heightened immune response, the body is less likely to recover from a major event, and chronic conditions follow.

Major events would include:

IMMUNE FUNCTION

- viral infection such as COVID-19, Epstein–Barr, glandular fever (mononucleosis), Lyme disease
- bacterial infection such as meningitis or major gut infections
- surgery including cosmetic surgery
- injury
- trauma
- big hormonal change
- immunization.

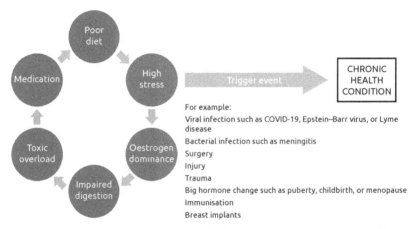

DIAGRAM 19 – CHRONIC HEALTH CAUSATION SHOWING HOW HEALTH AND LIFESTYLE ISSUES PARTNERED WITH A TRIGGER EVENT LEAD TO A CHRONIC HEALTH SITUATION

TAKE-HOME MESSAGE

Immune function is directly affected by the health and balance of our hormones. At a time of hormonal imbalance, it is imperative to keep digestive function optimal, blood sugars balanced, and stress under control; otherwise, inflammation and symptoms in the immune system can develop. We often see chronic conditions such as autoimmune disease and cancer develop over several years due to poor diet and high stress. For a woman heading into perimenopause or post-menopause, it is vitally important to keep the Triangle of Hormonal Health balanced to avoid triggering one of these outcomes and to support the management of existing conditions.

— CHAPTER 9 —

Putting the Triangle of Hormonal Health together

We've looked at each set of hormones, and now it's time to put them together so you can see how they layer to create the health picture that women are struggling with.

The women we see commonly have headaches, indigestion and IBS, hip pain, period/hormone issues (prior to and during menopause), anxiety, depression, overwhelm, thyroid imbalances, exhaustion, insomnia, high blood pressure, weight problems, allergies, intolerances, and autoimmune conditions...and perimenopause.

This is a standard list, and it's a lot for one person to be dealing with.

But this is the perfect example of a triangle that is out of balance, and as we have explored, millions of people, not just women, are walking around with bodies flooded with insulin, cortisol, and oestrogen.

And the first thing we look at is diet. Because getting that right will eliminate a lot of those symptoms. Then we can look at stress, address the fluctuating perimenopause hormones, and, if necessary, look at the gut and immune system. Commonly, these victims can improve once the foundations are back in place.

The following ladder looks at all the hormones we have talked about in the previous chapters so you can see the pathway to how these symptoms are created.

The base of this pyramid is diet and food intolerances because as we've said before, these are the foundations for health. When we are consistent with making poor choices in this base layer, we have cracks that show all the way up to the top of the pyramid.

This isn't about being perfect or the occasional time we go out binge drinking, this is about the decisions we make day in, day out for years that are contributing to blood sugar imbalances and stress, and ultimately more stress, and issues with hormones, gut, and our immune system.

10	Histamine intolerance, increased oestrogen, allergies
9	Chronic inflammation, high LDL, cholesterol, joint/muscle pain, and autoimmunity
8	Poor oestrogen detoxing, headaches, migranes
7	Intestinal permeability, infections, rashes, itching, bloating
6	Slowed gut function, motilin, constipation, IBS, continuous fatigue, and no energy
5	Progesterone deficiency, insomnia, depression, overwhelm, brain fog
4	Oestrogen increases, weight gain on breasts and glutes, menstrual cycle changes
3	Adrenaline spikes, raised cortisol, raised aldosterone, high blood pressure, fluid retention, feeling anxious, palpitations
2	Fluctuating blood sugar hormones, insulin spikes, high leptin, low ghrelin, CCK imbalance, sugar cravings, increased appetite, weight gain around the middle and arms, hyperglycemia
1	Poor diet – dehydration, stimulants, high carb, food intolerances, and ultra-processed food

DIAGRAM 20 – THE TRIANGLE OF HORMONAL HEALTH STACKING EFFECT SHOWING HOW DIET, LIFESTYLE, AND HORMONAL CHANGES CAN COMPOUND TOGETHER

This is a truly whole-health approach. It removes the bias towards quick fixes and focuses on getting back to eating and living in the way we evolved to eat and live, in a species-appropriate manner without ultra-processed food, cortisol-induced lifestyle choices, and medication that has a myriad of side effects. Taking control of our hormones means we are less reliant on big pharma, big food corporations interested in profit over health, and a medical system that is failing and under-resourced.

In a world that is creating an environment that promotes ill health and hormone destabilization from every single angle, the ultimate revolution is to live well.

And in Part Two, we are going to show you exactly how to do that.

— PART TWO —

How can I make my menopause better?

— CHAPTER 10 —

Menopause is a gift
– no, really…

The picture we have painted is a sombre one of women's bodies not coping with their environments, with autoimmune disease and insulin resistance being rife, a medical system that isn't focused on patient care, and cancer now being diagnosed in every other person. In 1993, Britpop band Blur proclaimed, "Modern Life is Rubbish." We can assure them that 30 years later things have not improved.

But this isn't the whole picture. We now have far more education and information to be able to make empowered informed decisions and take back control of our health. And we are now talking openly about menopause, hopefully ensuring that women can get the support they need.

Menopause is a gift. For women who are really struggling, we appreciate that this seems unlikely, but let us reframe it for you.

Many of us go through our lives putting other people first. We are taught to be good girls and people pleasers, where boundaries are commonly an alien concept in case we rock the boat or upset people. Then we have careers and children, and we get busy – very busy. And when we are busy, we often don't have time to prepare nourishing meals for ourselves and instead grab things on the run. We might not prioritize exercise or self-care. We don't have time for self-reflection and for stillness.

In popular culture, there is much discussion around the "four phases of womanhood". This is based on the "Triple Goddess" of the ancient pagan matriarchal tradition. Because modern women have longer lives, an extra phase has been added in more recent times. The phases are a great tool to help women understand what is happening, not just during menopause but during our whole life.

The "four phases of woman" is a way of explaining what is happening during each week of our cycle using archetypes and seasons, but if we look at the analogy in a broader context, it also explains the overarching life stages of a woman.

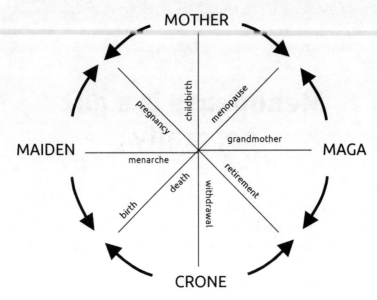

DIAGRAM 21 – THE MAGA WHEEL – THE STAGES OF A WOMAN'S LIFE REPRESENTED AS ARCHETYPES

First, we will look at it in the context of a monthly cycle and how, each week of the month, our mood and energy shift. If you are a woman who has experienced hormone imbalances, you may not have experienced the hormone cycle as it is meant to be, but instead had more of a rollercoaster. This is a map of how a woman with balanced hormones might feel.

Spring is the week after we have bled. The archetype of spring is **the Maiden**. We have lots of energy and the energy points outward. We feel more sociable and joyful.

Summer is the week of ovulation. We feel juicy and in full bloom; we are sexually more interested and easily aroused, and we are calm and happy. This is the archetype of **the Mother**. We have lots of tolerance, we are caring, and again our abundant energy is pouring outward.

Autumn is the week pre-bleed. The archetype here is **the Maga** (pronounced "maah-ga"), which translates as sorceress or high priestess. She is mysterious and powerful, and she has a fierce quality to her. Saying the wrong thing to her will mean she will give you back unfiltered truth. But this comes with incredible self-assurance because she knows who she is.

Her energy is starting to decline, so she is still sociable but less likely to want to go out. She is less caring about other people's thoughts and opinions, and, in this place of decline, she will assess conversations from a few weeks back. If we are people pleasing and being overly tolerant and brushing things aside, they often come back up to be discussed and worked through as our hormones change.

Interestingly, this is when we commonly say women are in "PMT"; it's too easy to give this a title just because we are more challenging and less amenable. We argue with our partners more, often over stupid things. We jokingly like to call this being "dishwasher-proportionate" (instead of disproportionate) because we will bite our partner's or children's head off for not emptying the dishwasher. The truth is, it isn't about the dishwasher; it's about the time they disrespected us or said something a few weeks ago, but we had too many caretaking hormones to notice then, and in the past few weeks the issue has sat and festered and turned into a resentment that needs clearing.

This is a very cleansing and powerful time. It is a time when we can find a lot of truth about situations if we learn to not beat ourselves up for not being "nice".

To be clear, we also believe that it is essential to learn some techniques around non-violent communication, so we aren't shouting or being passive-aggressive and creating an environment of abuse.

Our hormone ratios change every two and a half days through the menstrual cycle. The change in hormones brings with it a fluctuating effect with our perspective on the world and our emotional reactions. All these emotions are valid and make us the fascinating, deep, complex, fierce, and mysterious individuals we are. But society has taught us to filter and regulate, to be nice and more "genteel", which is completely at odds with our natural instincts. In the natural world, in almost every other species, it is the female that is to be feared. In the famous words of Rudyard Kipling, "The female of the species is more deadly than the male."

It is the combination of the mother as the protector and the Maga that fuels our ferocity when we allow ourselves to be who we truly are.

Winter is the week of our bleed. The energy of this time is internalized and low; it is dreamlike and self-reflective. This is the archetype of **the Crone**.

Historically, women have been considered deeply powerful and mysterious at this stage; our dreams and intuition are often heightened, but our desire to socialize (or rollerblade) is limited. Instead, we crave stillness and comfort.

"Wintering" is a practice we teach women who are struggling with their cycles, harking back to a time when women were given time away from their duties of cooking and caretaking. This was because they were considered "unclean". Now, of course, we see this as an incredibly discriminatory view, but the chance for a week of self-care and rest was valid. We teach women that even if it's just for an hour, it is important to have

Four phases as a lifecycle

Let's now revisit each of the four phases using the overarching theme of the whole lifecycle of a woman.

Spring – the Maiden: While there is no definitive age associated with each phase, a close approximation would be that Spring would take a woman through puberty up until her early 20s. During this time, our energy is external, and we are out in the world trying to figure it all out.

Summer – the Mother: Here is when we move from the "green naivety" of youth and start to embrace ourselves and develop our self-awareness. If we choose not to have children or are unable to have them, this fertile time is often when our careers take off and we are creating our homes. Again, our energy is outward, focusing on all these different areas in our life. This can be considered the mid-20s to early 40s.

Autumn – the Maga: This could be around a woman's early 40s to late 50s. This is an incredibly powerful and sexy time because we know ourselves deeply as a woman. Now is the time we use the deep intuition of the Maga to tune in to our life, work out what isn't serving us, and stop it. We find our boundaries; we stop putting everyone else first, and we step into our absolute authenticity. This powerful time in a woman's life is when she is a potent version of herself. We are usually at the peak of our career, and often it is the time when a woman has left a long-term relationship and is searching for a new partner who can meet her as she is now.

This is the time of perimenopause. Because our hormones are declining, there are changes in our personality. Oestrogen and progesterone are "mothering" hormones; they enable us to have tolerance and patience, and be in the role of a caretaker. Without these, we aren't "worse" people; we are more boundaried, more intolerant of bulls**t, and we have less energy to put into others.

But this is also beautiful. We have no choice but to be in radical self-care. There is a stigma around being selfish, but the definition of selfish is to have less concern for others than we do for ourselves. Isn't that great? Aren't we taught to put on our own oxygen mask first, before helping others? It's just alien to us if our conditioning has taught us to put everyone else first and ignore our own needs.

The liminal space of perimenopause is highlighting to us all what we need to leave behind. This will be different for different women, but it could include toxic dynamics or situations and behaviours that our body can no longer handle, be it late nights, eating too much junk, wearing high heels, rushing around like a headless chicken...

But when we do leave behind the things that aren't serving us, we give others permission to do the same. This allows us to move further and further into authenticity, deepening the connection and love for ourselves, and, ultimately, the potential is to have deeper and more authentic connections with our loved ones. We also become fierce, but in a different way to when we are younger: it has more grounding and wisdom to it.

In this phase, we start pulling on a different way of processing the world. Our brain, which commonly works quite fast and uses logic and reaction in the first two phases, suddenly develops a different pace. It feels slower; recall becomes harder and words start to leave us. We use the term "brain fog" to describe it, but because our intuition is heightened, it means we are now processing through "knowing" instead of just logic. We are at a place in our life when our life experiences, combined with this knowing and a slower pace, mean we are developing some incredible wisdom.

This is also a time for grief and letting go of what was and being with what is true now. And it is also a time to give thanks because we made it this far. Our ancestors commonly died before they had the chance to go through menopause, and sadly, with the rates of autoimmune disease, cancers, and death in childbirth being so high, I'm sure most of us have friends who haven't made it here. The grief and gratitude is an important process before we enter the final stage.

Winter – the Crone: Historically, this was considered to be the most powerful phase of a woman's life. Today, this would translate as being around 60+. As our energy becomes completely internalized, we are moving even further away from logical knowledge into the deep knowing wisdom, intuition, and insights.

Hollywood and fairy tales have made the crone an ugly wicked witch, but when we look at the dark history of female subjugation, we can see it is just as a woman is truly coming into her most powerful that we cut her down.

We only embrace women in their youth and in their mother phase, we don't embrace fierce women who are powerful and opinionated, perpetuating the belief that women are only beautiful when they are caretaking and people pleasing, and perfectly coiffed, plucked, nipped, tucked, and injected.

But older is also beautiful, in a different way.

The ultimate opportunity is to enter this stage of our life with ferocity. To find our "no", and to embrace our knowing as opposed to our knowledge.

Our perimenopause can therefore be a hugely transformational journey if we allow it to be, but we can't expect transformation without some growing pains. It is shining a light on what we must now look at *if* we are to transform.

And when we do this with courage and honesty, and we take a blowtorch to everything that is no longer serving us and step into the next phase of our life, claiming our "third age", we will not be the little old ladies who go quietly into our geriatric years. We will carry on being the fierce warrioresses who demanded more from their life and carved out new pathways for ourselves and for those who come after us.

But sometimes we need support to find that courage, to speak the truth and act on what we are facing. This is where practitioners, coaches, women's circles, retreats, and support groups can be incredibly helpful. Women are stronger together, and when we stand together collectively without comparison, judgement, and criticism, we have the power to change the course of history.

We hope that we have persuaded you that while this is a challenging time, it is also an important and potentially beautiful one. If we can bring this reframe around menopause being an important transformation, it is also easier to embrace the changes we need to make to our lifestyle, as they feel more like an act of self-love than a self-imposed restriction.

With the scene set, let's get honest about stressors and what we can do to reduce them.

— CHAPTER 11 —

How to reduce your stress(ors)

Biochemical stressors

The biochemical, electrical, emotional, and structural stressors that bombard us day in, day out are taking up our bandwidth. Some of these we can't do anything about. Unless we start walking around in a large bubble, we can't change the fact that we are exposed to pesticides, pollution, and radioactive particles every time we breathe.

But there are plenty of things in the stressor list that we can do something about. Making changes where we can frees up a lot of bandwidth, which means our body has more capacity to be able to buffer the rest.

But where do we start? We start as always with the things that we are exposed to every day, that have the biggest impact and are the easiest to tweak:

- food intolerances
- chemical toxicity
- clean water
- sleep hygiene
- exercise
- electromagnetic exposure
- getting into nature
- emotional issues
- structural issues.

Food intolerances

Food intolerances are common. The difference between an allergy and an intolerance is that an allergy will cause an immediate reaction such as vomiting, anaphylaxis, and hives, whereas an intolerance will cause milder symptoms between 20 minutes and four hours later. Example of these symptoms are gut pain, diarrhoea, fatigue, period issues, brain fog, bloating, itching, joint pain, headaches and migraines, and increased mucus (aka "the dairy snots").

Many of these symptoms can be overlooked or passed off as something else and not attributed to our diet. While many of these symptoms will pass, if we are exposed repeatedly to the food that is causing an intolerance, over time the symptom will develop or compound. Seemingly entrenched issues such as neck issues, sinus problems, knee or back pain, irritable bowel syndrome, and even carpal tunnel syndrome can be attributed to food intolerances and minimized when our exposure to foods we are intolerant to is reduced.

As we have previously explored, the intestinal permeability and immune reaction that happens in the presence of repeated food intolerance injury can also contribute to major chronic conditions such as autoimmune disease, diabetes, and even certain cancers.

There are reasons why we experience food intolerances. Some people experience more intolerances than others, and this is usually due to their health history and underlying immune issues and inflammation because of:

- poor digestive function

- microbiome dysbiosis such as SIBO and high histamine

- intestinal permeability

- stress and hormone instability

- choosing foods that are common sensitizers.

Food intolerances are important because they are a fundamental cause of destabilizing the Triangle of Hormonal Health.

When we eat food we are intolerant to, we have an adrenaline response, and it is this response that explains why we sometimes crave foods – we are literally adrenaline junkies looking for our next hit. Adrenaline and cortisol spike insulin, stop progesterone production, and disrupt the gut microbiome, which initiates an immune response. It's a perfect strike.

It is important to add here that food intolerances can lessen over time as digestive and immune function improve. However, if the digestion and immune functions worsen and hormones become more imbalanced, sensitivities can increase.

Foods that are common sensitizers

"Biochemical individuality" is a phrase often used in functional nutrition and kinesiology.

This is the technical term for the adage "one man's meat is another man's poison". Although we are all biochemically similar, we are very individual in how we respond to foods and environmental stressors.

Food intolerance testing has become popular. We aren't fans of many types of these tests because they only assess one type of immune response, which means a lot gets missed. It's also common to be sent a list of 60 foods that you are intolerant to without anyone assessing your diet and health history, and this can be overwhelming and unhelpful. They might show, for example, that kiwifruit are a major sensitizer for you, but you never eat kiwifruit, so you end up none the wiser on what is causing you a problem.

One of our favourite questions is "What are you eating every day?"

If you have symptoms, we must look at the obvious triggers.

Kinesiology food testing is brilliant for finding out what foods are specifically a problem for you as an individual and which foods are good for you, and a good kinesiologist will look at all the information about your health and diet and choose to test foods that are relevant to you.

But in the absence of a kinesiologist, you can work out your own triggers using our food intolerance hierarchy. People are usually surprised by which foods are common sensitizers.

What is the food intolerance hierarchy?

The food intolerance hierarchy is a process for eliminating food sensitizers based on the commonality of that food causing an issue.

The hierarchy has been created by fusing a variety of approaches such as the Autoimmune Protocol and the FODMAP diet. However, these diets tend to do a blanket elimination, which means we have no clarity on what is truly causing the issue, so we have created a step-by-step approach.

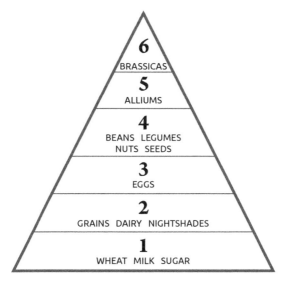

DIAGRAM 22 – THE FOOD INTOLERANCE HIERARCHY

Level 1 – the gateway allergens

The gateway allergens are the foundations of food intolerance issues and can contribute to (and even cause) a multitude of symptoms. These gateway allergens can create a generalized immune response. Many foods can be viewed as a problem, but our focus needs to be to eliminate the main problem foods.

Wheat, milk, and sugar are commonly consumed foods that lead to a huge amount of biochemical fallout in the body and can destabilize the Triangle of Hormonal Health every time they are eaten.

We call them the "gateway allergens" because sometimes people can be seemingly intolerant and even allergic to many things but are regularly consuming these three foods. For people with many allergies and intolerances, eating becomes riddled with anxiety as it will inevitably lead to symptom flare-ups and can be life-affecting. They may also be experiencing an escalation in symptoms such as hay fever and reactions to washing powders and toiletries. It can feel as though they are becoming allergic to the whole world.

The truth is that the three gateway allergen foods are causing a lot of underlying immune and digestive impairment, which in turn causes widespread inflammation. This means that for some, their body starts to overreact to anything and everything. It's not a clear picture: the underlying digestive and immune impairments are muddying the water.

When these three gateway allergens are eliminated, the digestive and immune systems can regulate and stop overreacting. Bit by bit, we then stop having unpredictable reactions and intolerances. Even full-blown allergies change as our immune response normalizes.

Of course, these are foods we have often been exposed to from the moment we are weaned. The damage to our gut caused by these foods can last a lifetime.

When talking about food intolerances (or any stressor), we use the phrase "dose and exposure" – how much of the food are you having and how often?

In the case of wheat, milk, and sugar, the standard Western diet can be full of them, and it can be considered normal for someone to be exposed to them four or five times a day.

An example would be:

- toast and Weetabix/bran flakes with milk and sugar for breakfast

- biscuit or wheat-based snack with a cup of tea/coffee and milk

- sandwich and chocolate or baked goods for lunch

- cake or wheat-based snack with a cup of tea/coffee and milk

- pasta, pizza, or breaded products (e.g. breaded fish) and yogurt with fruit for dinner

- a cup of milky tea and a biscuit before bed.

That is a lot of exposure to foods causing your body to be under stress and requiring an immune response.

We have lost count of the number of times we have worked with clients who are seemingly complicated cases with major issues. Many of them have worked with expensive nutritionists and practitioners but they are still consuming the gateway allergens.

Once they've given these up, often within weeks they feel completely different.

CASE STUDY: "SARAH", 44

Symptoms: Shortness of breath, intense brain fog, and debilitating fatigue.

History: Doctors have been querying long COVID, asthma, and perimenopause.

Assessment: It could be any of these things, but her diet leads us to believe that food intolerances are playing a part in this picture, possibly exacerbated by early perimenopause.

Her diet consists of:

- breakfast: cereal with added protein powder

- lunch: protein source with sweet potato mash and root vegetables

- takeaways at the weekend

- dinner: Meat and vegetables

- snacks: KitKat or similar.

This type of diet seems quite typical – in fact, compared to many, it's got quite a lot of proper meals, but there is also a possibility that wheat, milk, and sugar are in her diet up to four times a day some days.

But why are these three foods so problematic?

Wheat

Back in the 1950s, wheat was an expensive and nutritious commodity. It was also not very resistant to pests, and it was top-heavy, so crops could be easily spoiled.

By the 1960s, an American agronomist called Dr Norman Borlaug had created a wheat hybrid that was semi-dwarf, high-yield, and very disease-resistant. He won a Nobel Peace Prize for this work as it was considered that he saved a billion people from dying from starvation.

While the modification worked to create a more resistant crop, a side effect was that the gluten content was dramatically increased.

Gluten is a protein that we cannot digest. The undigested protein triggers the immune system to attack the lining of the small intestine. Although this elevated gluten on its own was highly problematic, the issue became compounded in the 1980s with the introduction and widespread use of a herbicide called glyphosate (aka Roundup).

Glyphosate has been linked to major health issues and has now been banned in many countries. It has a massive impact on the bacteria in the gut. It interrupts the production of "happy brain chemicals" serotonin and dopamine. It also reduces our ability to process fructose, which then gets stored as fat, creates a fatty liver, increases cholesterol, and impairs the body's ability to eliminate toxins.

The combination of higher gluten content in the grain and glyphosate destroys the effectiveness of our gut microbiome and our metabolism.

The Western world now has a diet dominated by wheat. It is in everything: bran, pasta, bread, bagels, desserts, and cereals, and it is often used as filler. It is cheap, easy to manufacture, and has a long shelf life. Modern wheat is not nutritious; in fact, it has a reduced mineral content compared to the original grain. It also contains preservatives that are immune stimulators, and it is usually processed to remove the bran and the wheat germ.

As well as the gluten and glyphosate, wheat naturally contains two types of plant compounds which are part of the plant's protection mechanism to stop predators from eating them. These compounds have been shown to cause problems to our health.

The first is lectins. When consumed, lectins aggravate and damage our gut lining. The second is phytates. Phytates are "antinutrients", which means they actively stop you absorbing certain vitamins and minerals.

The plain truth is, whichever way you look at it, modern wheat is poison. We liken it to arsenic and often ask the question "How much arsenic do you think you could have in your diet before you felt unwell?"

We are commonly asked if brown bread is better than white – the answer is that both are arsenic.

We are asked if organic wheat is OK – the answer is that it's still arsenic because of the high gluten; it's just arsenic that hasn't been sprayed with glyphosate.

We also get asked if sourdough is OK – the answer is that sourdough is just fermented arsenic.

There is no way around it. If we want to be well, we must ditch the wheat. For good.

Cow's milk

The presence of cow's milk among the gateway allergens is often a surprise to many people. After all, humans have a long-standing belief that cow's milk is an essential and healthy food. Like wheat, we wean our children on it, and we can be exposed to it multiple times in a day.

But also, like wheat, modern milk production is a far cry from the wholesome image we may be able to conjure up of the sound of cow bells in the Swiss mountains or a traditional British farm with a jug of fresh milk on the kitchen table.

The aggressive modern farming system is particularly brutal when it comes to the dairy industry. Repeated artificial insemination, separation of mothers from their calves, cows with mastitis, widespread use of antibiotics, hormones, and feed that isn't species appropriate, followed by pasteurization and homogenization means that "the White Stuff" is incredibly inflammatory and insulinogenic.

There are multiple reasons why milk can cause an issue.

Lactose intolerance is a sensitivity to the sugar lactose in dairy products and is caused by not having the enzyme lactase to break it down. Changing to lactose-free milk is only part of the picture, however. This milk has been even more processed to remove the lactose, and people are often just as intolerant to other aspects of milk.

Casein is one of the proteins in milk. There are four types of casein, but we only need to talk about two of them here: as-1 casein (casein 1) and as-2 casein (casein 2). Some animals such as sheep and goats (and some breeds of cow) produce milk that predominantly contains casein 2. This casein is much easier for humans to digest as it's the dominant protein in human breast milk. Multiple studies have found that the regular consumption of casein 1 is linked to type 1 and type 2 diabetes, heart disease, respiratory conditions, and digestive upset.

Milk contains "protease inhibitors" that neutralize our digestive enzymes.

However, an enzyme called trypsin is increased in response to milk consumption; this enzyme can contribute to breaking down the bonds between cells, leading to intestinal permeability.

Milk is very insulinogenic due to its sweetness, especially semi-skimmed and skimmed milk.

Due to the farming methods involved, milk has elevated levels of oestrogen, progesterone, and cortisol, which mess up our own hormone signalling and hormone metabolism.

Raw milk is gaining in popularity, especially raw milk with casein 2 as it contains excellent fats and vitamins, but it is often not a case of swapping to this type of milk (if you are lucky enough to be able to source it). We usually have to give the body a period without milk entirely to reduce the inflammation and for the immune response to change.

There is a popular belief that the acid created by consuming dairy products reduces the calcium in our bones. Whether this is true or not is difficult to ascertain as there are as many websites showing the evidence as there are disproving it, but what we do know is that pasteurized dairy is hard to digest and stimulates the mucous membranes, which is an inflammatory response. If we have symptoms, it needs to be removed from our diets.

Sugar

The negative effects of processed sugar are well documented and include obesity, heart disease, diabetes, inflammation, gut dysbiosis, increased pressure on the pancreas, endocrine disorders, and a fatty liver. We all know that too much sugar is bad for us, but the problem is that, again, it is in so many foods that it can be hard to avoid.

Part of the reason for this is obfuscation. Sugar goes by many different names. These include fructose, sucrose, glucose, dextrose, galactose, maltodextrin, mannitol, and sorbitol, but there are many more. Not to mention the pervasive and dangerous high-fructose corn syrup. These "hidden" sugars are often found in many processed foods.

Sugar is highly addictive – some sources claim it is as addictive as cocaine. Once we have some of the underlying conditions such as diabetes or gut dysbiosis, the hormonal fluctuations they create can distort our behaviours, meaning we keep reaching for the sugar.

"Food addiction" is now a term being bandied around in many medical spheres, where they see a correlation between these distorted behaviours and a high-carbohydrate diet. Food addiction hasn't been officially classed as an addiction yet, but many coaches who work with diet and doctors trying to deal with diabetes are seeing how hard it can be to break the behaviours associated with high-sugar diets.

This is a relatively new problem. In the 1700s, sugar was very expensive and mostly bought by the very wealthy, and now our daily intake has dramatically escalated.

When you consider that the human body evolved by eating seasonal fruit that was found in our environment, honey, and root vegetables, it is clear to see that we are not designed to metabolize this much sugar.

Much of our sugar now comes in the form of high-fructose corn syrup which is used to sweeten foods like ketchup and fizzy drinks. It is incredibly dangerous for humans as it contains large amounts of fructose, and the liver is the only organ that can metabolize fructose in significant amounts. When your liver gets overloaded, it turns the fructose into fat and stores it, contributing to fatty liver. High fructose consumption is also linked to insulin resistance, metabolic syndrome, obesity, and type 2 diabetes. The other issue is that because this syrup is often in drinks, which don't spend much time in the mouth being chewed, our body doesn't get enough time to produce the insulin required to deal with it before it hits our bloodstream. A huge sugar spike without the hormones to handle it is a problem. Substitutes that sound like healthier versions of this, such as agave nectar, are still just high-fructose syrups and best avoided.

As well as the obvious blood sugar destabilizing effects, sugar is also linked to an increase in autoimmunity and some cancers. It is imperative that we reduce sugar consumption if we are going to reduce the stress on our body and rebalance our hormones.

What about sweeteners?

Sweeteners are also a bit of a minefield, and some, such as aspartame, saccharin, and acesulfame, are well documented to be highly toxic.

These sweeteners imitate sugar, the body reacts as if sugar has been consumed by producing insulin, but when no real sugar comes, then the body must counteract the high insulin, and we tend to eat more to bring down these levels. This is therefore creating an entirely unnecessary blood sugar rollercoaster, and the upshot is insulin resistance, weight gain, and poor blood sugar management for diabetics.

These sweeteners are also highly inflammatory and linked to a variety of conditions including autoimmune diseases and fibromyalgia.

Sucralose is the most popular sweetener in the world, commonly known by its brand name Splenda. It has, however, also been linked to diabetes, Crohn's disease, IBS, intestinal permeability, and weight gain. It is also a known carcinogen.

Xylitol and erithyritol are often touted as being the healthier options.

These sweeteners are called "sugar alcohols", which is quite confusing as they aren't alcohol.

Although it's true that they don't spike blood sugars and so are better for blood sugar management, and they contain fewer calories than sugar, there are multiple reasons to avoid them.

These sugar alcohols can't be digested, which means we can't utilize them. This in turn can cause quite a few issues, mostly with our digestion. These sweeteners are notorious for causing loose bowels as they have a laxative effect. While some studies show that 10–15 grams a day is a safe dose, others show that erythritol is closely associated with an increased risk of major cardiovascular events including heart attack and stroke.

One definite benefit of xylitol, however, is that it is very good for teeth and stops harmful bacteria that can contribute to cavities.

Many schools of thought say that these "sugar alcohols" have no place in a whole-food diet; however, as an interim measure to wean people off refined sugar, they can be useful when used moderately.

What can I use?

Stevia or steviol glycoside is a natural sweetener from the stevia plant and has been used as a sweetener for thousands of years. It is commercially available in liquid or crystal form. When it is processed, it is also a sugar alcohol. Used in moderation, it doesn't seem to cause as much of an issue as the others, but the research isn't available for us to be sure. Again, occasional use seems to be fine.

There are some beneficial sweeteners.

As with everything dietary related, the more we go back to nature, the better it is for us. The most beneficial sweeteners are:

Raw, unfiltered honey: This is the kind of honey you would buy from a farm shop that has been harvested by local beekeepers. This is an important distinction because most commercial honey is boiled (including most Manuka honeys) and therefore becomes a high-fructose syrup and brings with it the negative health effects mentioned previously. Raw honey is a perfectly balanced carbohydrate and contains nitric oxide which stabilizes our blood sugar and contributes to vascular health.

Pure maple syrup: Again, making sure that the maple syrup is real and not a syrup substitute is important because real maple syrup has multiple benefits such as being rich in antioxidants, vitamins, and minerals, and having a lesser impact on blood sugars than sugar. However, it is recommended to be moderate with any sweetener if you have diabetes.

Blackstrap molasses: Packed full of vitamins and minerals including iron, blackstrap molasses is a traditional sweetener that doesn't spike blood sugars.

Coconut sugar: This is the sugar from coconut tree resin. It is a balanced sugar that also contains good fats and a fibre called inulin, which is good for the gut. However, honey or blackstrap molasses are preferred if you have diabetes as coconut sugar has more of a destabilizing effect on blood sugars.

> **TAKE-HOME MESSAGE**
> Avoiding the gateway allergens – wheat, dairy, and sugar – is essential if we want to get our hormones balanced and get back our health and vitality.

We recommend giving up these foods for a month and seeing what impact it has on your symptoms.

If you still have symptoms, it's time to take the next step up the ladder of the hierarchy of food intolerances.

Level 2 – Other grains, dairy and nightshades

Other grains

For all the reasons previously discussed, wheat really is problematic. For many people, it is enough to eliminate it from the diet to be able to experience symptom relief.

However, for others, we need to go further and remove all grains.

This is commonly due to something called "gluten cross-sensitivity" where the immune system sees something that looks a bit like wheat and reacts as if it *is* wheat. It is possible over time that this cross-sensitivity will stop once the immune system is less reactive. However, many researchers have documented the negative effects of grains on our health.

Grains including spelt, rye, oats, and barley:

- spike blood sugar insulin levels

- are not a good source of fibre due to being an intestinal irritant

- contain sticky proteins and antinutrients that are the plant's way of protecting itself – these damage gut lining and increase permeability

- are small and hard to digest

- damage gut lining and permeability

- increase inflammation

- contribute to leptin resistance, affecting hunger levels

- contain phytates.

This is contrary to much of the marketing and conditioning that tells us grains are good for us. Porridge is hailed as a perfect breakfast, but for many people struggling with symptoms, this is simply not true.

Dairy

We add dairy separately to milk as for many people, removing cow's milk in 'milk form' from their diet is enough to make changes to their symptoms and they can enjoy cheese, yogurt and cream as nutritious contributors to their diet. However, for other people it is necessary to go further and remove other dairy items. Dairy can stimulate oestrogen and contribute to inflammation and this is problem for many people.

Nightshades

Members of the nightshade family are, to many people, truly deadly. Their appearance in the hierarchy often comes as a surprise because these are also foods that we would consider "healthy" – one of our "five a day" and safe and good because they are vegetables. However, tomatoes, potatoes, aubergines, peppers, and chillies are other insidious, potentially toxic ingredients that make an appearance in many staple daily dishes.

The nightshade family contains chemicals called saponins and alkaloids, and they also have lectins. All these chemicals are designed to protect the plant from consumption; again, they cross the gut barrier, triggering an immune response.

They also hinder the growth of some beneficial probiotic bacteria and stimulate the overgrowth of those pesky gram-negative bacteria. On top of that, the saponins also bind to fat-soluble vitamins, meaning we don't absorb them, so they act as an antinutrient.

One of Claire's favourite stories about nightshades is from her own journey. Having experienced hospitalization from migraines repeatedly in her early teens, Claire had to take a non-steroidal anti-inflammatory medication daily. When she was learning about food testing in 2007, her kinesiology class was asked to bring in their favourite foods. Claire had been a huge fan of tomatoes since she was a toddler, and they featured heavily in her diet, both raw and cooked. Barely a day went by when she wouldn't eat them.

When she found out during the class that she was intolerant to them, she was devastated but decided to try removing them from her diet.

Within two weeks, a lot had changed. She lost a stone in weight without changing anything else except avoiding tomatoes. After a month, she realized she hadn't had a headache, and she came off her medication; since then, she has had less than a handful of migraines and certainly nothing like the visual migraines she had before.

Headaches, migraines, postnasal drip, IBS, skin rashes, heartburn, indigestion, reflux, allergies, haemorrhoids, anal fissures, and bowel issues are associated with nightshade foods, and eliminating them can be a game changer. But if you are still having symptoms after a few weeks, it's time to proceed to level 3.

Level 3 – Eggs[1]

Eggs are a valuable food, high in protein, fat, and essential nutrients.

However, for some people with sensitive guts and a reactive immune system, they can contribute to a lot of symptoms.

Egg whites contain a protein which is an enzyme called lysozyme. Lysozyme is essentially an antimicrobial to keep the yolk protected. However, this protection also means that it wards off predators from eating them.

Lysozyme stops the egg white from being digested properly; when it encounters the gut, it can cross the gut barrier. This "leak" then allows other egg white proteins through the gut wall into the bloodstream, triggering an immune response.

Very sensitive people often find they can tolerate the yolks better than the whites, but, again, it may take some time for the immune system to calm down and be able to tolerate any part of the egg.

You guessed it...if this hasn't caused all your symptoms to abate, it's time to move to Level 4.

Level 4 – Beans, legumes, nuts, and seeds

Beans and legumes are high-FODMAP foods. FODMAP stands for fermentable oligosaccharides, disaccharides, monosaccharides, and polyols. They are specific carbohydrates that are known to trigger IBS and other bowel conditions as they absorb a lot of water and are hard to digest, so they can ferment in the bowel.

They are also high in lectins like grains, and they contain oxalates, a naturally occurring compound in plants that binds to calcium and increases the risk of kidney stones.

Many people find symptomatic relief when they are removed from the diet.

Nuts and seeds are another surprising entry in the food intolerance hierarchy. They contain lectins, which irritate the gut, and oxalates. They also contain a substance called phytate. Phytates contain phytic acid which can contribute to anaemia and zinc, magnesium, and calcium deficiency.

Nuts are also high in omega 6. While omega 3 is very beneficial, omega 6 is inflammatory and can lead to elevated blood pressure, issues with blood sugar balancing, and water retention.

Those with sensitive digestions may struggle to digest nuts, especially with the brown skins on, as these are a defence mechanism designed to make them indigestible.

What many people don't know about nuts is that although they are considered a "good fat", they can also contribute to retaining weight. The fat in nuts is called linoleic acid. Linoleic acid signals to our fat cells to hold on to fat because "winter is coming" due to the historic seasonality of when we would have eaten them. (In contrast, meat fat contains stearic acid and due to our ancestry of being hunters, when we consume stearic acid, our fat cells get the message that there is an abundance of food, so it is safe to go into fat-burning mode.)

And if you've eliminated all these things and are still experiencing symptoms, we need to go to level 5.

Level 5 – Alliums
Alliums include onions, shallots, chives, spring onions, garlic, and leeks. This group are high-FODMAP foods and contribute to digestive upset.
Last and by no means least, if there is still inflammation or symptoms that you can't clear, it's time to face the hard truth that kale doesn't love you back.

Level 6 – Brassicas
Brassicas include broccoli, cabbage, cauliflower, rapeseed, mustard, kohlrabi, bok choi, turnip, kale, purple kale, Brussel sprouts, collard greens, and rutabaga.

Yes, we know that this goes against everything we've ever been taught about eating our greens, but there is a growing body of research and an expanding community of thought leaders and health advocates who are opposed to this belief. Us included. It took some serious processing when we realized that broccoli wasn't our friend.

Remember this is Level 6 in the food hierarchy, so you are only eliminating these foods if all else fails, but, for many people (us included), removing these foods can have a huge impact on improving symptoms.

The reason brassicas can be a problem is that while plants generally want us to eat their fruit, they don't want us to eat their seeds, leaves, stems, and roots because this would be detrimental to their survival. These elements therefore contain chemicals to deter animals from eating them. These chemicals include sulforaphane, oxalates, and isothiocyanates (which are compounds made from cyanide).

These chemicals can affect your thyroid and hormones and can be a major trigger for autoimmune flare-ups and inflammation, so while it may seem extreme, eliminating these foods can be hugely beneficial.

The 14 common allergens

We must also remember that there are 14 allergens that are so common that they must be listed on food packaging. These are: gluten (such as wheat, barley, and oats), crustaceans (such as prawns, crabs, and lobsters), celery, eggs, fish, lupin, milk, molluscs (such as mussels and oysters), mustard, peanuts, sesame, soybeans, sulphur dioxide, and sulphites.

When you consider the list of foods in the food intolerance hierarchy and then the 14 common allergens and how often we may consume these foods (sometimes up to five times a day!), you can see why food intolerance is a major contributor to stress in the body.

Ultra-processed foods and seed oils

Although they aren't included in the food intolerance hierarchy or the common allergens list, it would be remiss of us not to mention ultra-processed foods and seed oils, as these are now being reported as being major contributors to poor health.

Ultra-processed foods include packaged baked goods and snacks, fizzy drinks, sugary cereals, ready meals containing food additives, dehydrated vegetable soups, and reconstituted meat and fish products – often containing high levels of added sugar, fat, and salt. These foods are lacking in vitamins and fibre. The intake of these foods has escalated dramatically, and the UK is currently the world leader in the consumption of ultra-processed foods.

While studies originally linked them to weight gain, obesity, and diabetes, emerging research is showing the connection between these foods and high blood pressure, high cholesterol, cardiovascular disease, and some cancers.

Seed oils have had a lot of column inches recently. The consumption of these oils has also escalated, and these industrial oils – also known as vegetable oil – are in nearly everything. If we use common cooking oils, eat pre-packaged foods, or dine out at restaurants, we can be exposed to them often.

In the 100 years since the processing of seed oils was established, we have seen increases in a variety of symptoms, and they have been linked to obesity, diabetes, heart disease, and cancer.

These oils include canola oil, corn oil, cottonseed oil, soy oil, sunflower oil, grapeseed oil, safflower oil, and rice bran oil, many of which have been wrongly categorized as healthy. The creation of them requires industrial processing, which couldn't be further removed from a natural whole-food diet.

If you are thinking, "What *can* I eat?" – don't panic. We are going into that in depth in Chapter 13.

But now, let's move on to the next item on the stressors list.

Chemical toxicity

Chemical toxicity is the build-up of chemicals we get from exposure to pesticides, pollution, home air fresheners, domestic cleaning products, toiletries, cosmetics, and perfumes.

Again, some of these we cannot control, like pesticides and pollution, but we can control what we put on our skin and clean our homes with.

The average woman is exposed to up to 50 products a day, which means there is exposure to up to 500 different chemicals in that 24-hour period. This is important when we consider that 60 per cent of the chemicals we put on our skin get absorbed into the body.

Often, it's not any one product that is the problem. It's the combination of many products, all containing cheap and toxic chemicals which, when combined, can have chemical interferences.

There are numerous studies to show that the synthetic chemicals in toiletries and cosmetics disrupt the endocrine system.[2]

There are hundreds of problem chemicals, but we focus on removing what we call the Big Six!

Paraffin (aka petroleum jelly or petrolatum)

This is one of the main offenders in skin issues. It is literally everywhere and seems to appear in almost every product. It is a hydrocarbon derived from crude oil, like petrol (hence the name). It's also known as a mineral oil, and its commercial purpose is to create "slip". It is a major skin disruptor. It lies like a layer of grease on the skin, stopping the skin's respiratory function and disrupting the skin's natural moisturizing mechanisms. Imagine you were wearing latex gloves all day every day. The sweat would come out of your skin, but it couldn't go anywhere, so you'd end up with your skin being all soggy but unable to breathe.

Over time, the skin's natural moisturising mechanisms are ruined; we stop being able to regulate this natural function and skin dries out permanently. This process also leads to rashes, increased chapping (usually the very thing we are using it to stop), and, worse, premature ageing! On top of the skin issues, a study by the University of Columbia showed that women with breast cancer were 2.6 times more likely to have these hydrocarbons in their DNA.[3]

Propylene glycol

Also labelled as PEG or PPG, this is another petrochemical derivative, and it is commercially used in the following ways:

- as a solvent, which helps one ingredient dissolve into another, producing a solution

- as a stabilizer, helping to keep products constant at various temperatures

- as an emulsifier, which helps mix a variety of ingredients

- as a humectant, helping formulations to attract and hold on to moisture.

Propylene glycol sits on the surface of your skin in the same way petroleum does, slowly drying it out because it attracts and draws moisture from the lower layers into the top layer. This gives the effect of your skin appearing moisturized and smooth and soft, but over time those lower layers dry out. Propylene glycol also enhances penetration. That means the cream or lotion you're using is more likely to penetrate the surface layer of the skin, which we don't want when those creams contain chemicals like petroleum.

According to the Material Safety Data Sheet, it is a strong skin irritant, and has been implicated in contact dermatitis; it can inhibit skin cell growth and damage cell membranes, causing rashes and dry skin. It has also been linked to allergies and respiratory issues.[4]

Sodium laureth sulphate or sodium lauryl sulphate (SLS)

SLS is essentially an industrial degreaser. It strips grease and is responsible for causing "foam" in products that clean such as shampoo and shower gel.

We have a natural protective layer called the "acid mantle" on our skin and scalp. When the acid mantle is balanced, we have beautifully healthy skin and hair.

The acid mantle is slightly acidic, meaning it creates an unfavourable environment for bugs and bacteria. It is literally part of our skin's protective barrier and forms part of our immune system. The "acid" is made up of sebum and sweat and is a little bit oily.

SLS strips away the acid mantle, along with the protection it offers. It also strips our natural oils; over time, this not only makes our skin lacklustre but causes actual damage.

SLS is widely known to be responsible for dermatitis and inflammation. Scientifically, SLS is an environmental toxin as well as a problem for us.

Now, we need to be extra vigilant because often a product will advertise that their SLS comes from palm oil or coconuts. This is one of the "pseudo-natural" claims that we need to be alert to. The initial raw materials can either be from petroleum (again) or coconut/palm oil. Once it has been stripped, processed, and generally played around with, it makes no difference to the final product. SLS is SLS regardless of how it started its life, and it is still a highly toxic and damaging chemical.

Parabens

Parabens are chemical preservatives used to extend the life of the products. They are not just in cosmetics; they are in anything that needs preservatives – from food to flat-packed furniture.

You will see them on packaging with names like methylparaben, ethylparaben, propylparaben, and butylparaben. These are in a category of chemicals called EDCs, which stands for endocrine disruptor chemicals – which is why they need to be avoided at all costs.

In terms of symptoms, they are known to cause allergic reactions and skin rashes, but that is just the start of the problems they cause. Parabens are classified as xeno-oestrogens, which means they are one of the chemicals that mimic and increase oestrogen.

Whether they are the cause or not is unknown, but parabens are often found in breast cancer tumours. Often when people are diagnosed with breast cancer, they are advised to avoid products containing parabens (and deodorants containing aluminium). They have also been linked to fertility problems and genital birth defects in children (e.g. boys being born with the urethra on the side of the penis not on the end).

The increased use of parabens combined with growth hormones in meat has contributed to the average age of menarche dropping from 14 in the 1980s to 11 in 2016.

Now, a lot of companies will also use the get-out clause that they only use "water-soluble parabens" or "parabens from blueberries". While it is true that some foodstuffs contain naturally occurring chemicals that are like parabens, they are not the same as the ones that are used commercially, so it's a weak claim used by companies who just don't want to go to the expense of reformulating.

Parfum

The word "parfum" is an umbrella term. Companies are allowed to use up to 200 different chemicals without listing them individually and hide them under the word "parfum". The issue here is lack of transparency, so you can't establish what chemicals are hiding in here, and this could include skin irritants and EDCs.

Companies who are organic or clean will use the word "parfum" followed by a statement such as "derived from essential oils".

Phthalates

Phthalates (pronounced "thalates" with a silent "ph") are essentially a group of chemicals that are plasticizers: they make products more flexible and harder to break. They are also used to lubricate and help products penetrate the skin.

On labels they will be called things like DBP, DNOP, DiNP, DEP; the most famous is BPA, often found in plastic bottles and children's toys.

In toiletries, phthalates are found in products like hairspray and nail varnish. There is a huge list of side effects on the phthalates Wikipedia page, but in short, they have been found to be endocrine disruptors. They have been linked to obesity, fertility issues, increased stillbirths, and even extra ribs at birth.

It is important to note that marketing departments go to great lengths to hide these chemical nasties. Do not be fooled by the words "natural" or "contains organic". These are marketing ploys! Companies are allowed to say "contains natural ingredients" even if they only contain 1 per cent natural ingredients and 99 per cent toxic chemicals.

Although it's not in skincare, there is another substance we can try and avoid…

Per- and polyfluoroalkyl substances (PFAS)

Used in products like Teflon and stain-resistant carpets, PFASs are resistant to breakdown and are found in our soil and groundwater. For decades, chemical companies covered up the health risks of PFAS, which include cancer and other diseases. Today, virtually all of us, including newborn infants, have PFAS compounds in our blood. These "forever chemicals" are shown to suppress healthy immune function, create chronic inflammation, and contribute to conditions including autoimmune disorders. We can avoid them by finding alternatives to Teflon for our cooking equipment.

Clean water

Two litres of water a day is an essential part of our diet, and contrary to what the medical profession tells us, fruit juices, tea, coffee, and packet soups (what?!?) are not counted towards this requirement.

Dehydration is a huge stress on the body and contributes to many chronic health symptoms. About two-thirds of the human body is made of water so we need to replenish it daily with pure still water.

Carbonated water is made with carbon dioxide, which is the primary toxin the body is working to remove during respiration, so while we can use fizzy water as a treat, we need to ensure we are also having enough still water.

Tea and coffee are diuretics and cause us to urinate more frequently, meaning we cannot rely on the water in these kinds of drinks. Other drinks like juice or squash are seen by the body as food, and there is a hormone response to them.

Water has many functions, including:

- moistening tissues such as those in the mouth, eyes, nose, bowel, and vagina

- protecting body organs and tissues

- preventing constipation (40% of the water we drink is used by the bowel)

- regulating body temperature

- lubricating joints

- lessening the burden on the kidneys and liver by flushing out waste products

- providing the electrical "carrier" signals in the brain and nervous system, thereby supporting clear thinking and processing, and helping the brain to communicate with muscles

- dissolving minerals to make them available in the body

- carrying nutrients and oxygen to the cells.

While many of us are blessed to live in countries with taps that conveniently give us clean water, it is still advisable to filter it. Many chemicals and contaminants such as chlorine, limescale, microplastic, fluoride (in some places), traces of hormones from pill and HRT use, traces of other medications such as antidepressants, and stimulants such as caffeine and cocaine are often found in the water supply.

Because of the effect of plastics on our hormones, avoiding bottled water is a good idea. Instead, opt for a countertop filter jug or an under-the-sink filter.

Sleep hygiene

Getting good sleep is essential for reducing stress and allowing our body to regenerate. According to the CDC, one in three adults are sleep deprived.[5] We will never be able to enhance our bandwidth if we are tired.

Insomnia is a common symptom of menopause, and many women struggle with it, but we can help ourselves by practising good sleep hygiene.

Optimizing your sleep schedule, pre-bed routine, and daily routines is part of harnessing habits to make quality sleep feel more automatic.

Here are our sleep hacks:

Set your sleep schedule. Having a set schedule normalizes sleep as an essential part of your day and gets your brain and body accustomed to getting the full amount of sleep that you need.

Have a fixed wake-up time. Regardless of whether it's a weekday or weekend, try to wake up at the same time, since a fluctuating schedule keeps you from getting into a rhythm of consistent sleep.

Prioritize sleep. It might be tempting to skip sleep to work, study, socialize, or exercise, but it's vital to treat sleep as a priority. Calculate a target bedtime based on your fixed wake-up time and do your best to be ready for bed around that time each night.

Make gradual adjustments. If you want to shift your sleep times, don't try to do it in one fell swoop, because that can throw your schedule out of whack. Instead, make small, step-by-step adjustments of up to an hour at a time.

Don't over-nap. Naps can be a handy way to regain energy during the day, but they can throw off sleep at night. To avoid this, try to keep naps relatively short and limited to the early afternoon.

Follow a nightly routine. Preparing the same routine each night will help your body get ready for sleep.

Keep your routine consistent. Following the same steps each night, including things like putting on your pyjamas and brushing your teeth, can reinforce in your mind that it's bedtime.

Allow 30 minutes for winding down. Take advantage of whatever puts you in a state of calm, such as soft music, light stretching, reading, or relaxation exercises.

Dim your lights. Try to keep away from bright lights because they can hinder the production of melatonin, a hormone that the body creates to facilitate sleep.

Unplug from electronics. Build in a 30–60-minute pre-bed buffer time that is device-free. Phones, tablets, and laptops cause mental stimulation that is hard to shut off and generate blue light that may decrease melatonin production.

Test methods of relaxation. Instead of making falling asleep your goal, it's often easier to focus on relaxation. Meditation, mindfulness, paced breathing, and other relaxation techniques can put you in the right mindset for bed. If your mind is whirring, try journaling.

Don't toss and turn. It helps to have a healthy mental connection between being in bed and being asleep. For that reason, if you haven't fallen asleep after 20 minutes, get up and stretch, read, or do something else calming in low light before trying to fall asleep again.

Get daylight exposure. Light, especially sunlight, is one of the key drivers of circadian rhythms that can encourage quality sleep.

Be physically active. Regular exercise can make it easier to sleep at night and delivers a host of other health benefits.

Reduce alcohol consumption. Alcohol may make it easier to fall asleep, but the effect wears off, disrupting sleep later in the night. As a result, it's best to moderate alcohol consumption and avoid it later in the evening.

Cut down on caffeine in the afternoon and evening. Because it's a stimulant, caffeine can keep you wired even when you want to rest, so try to avoid it later in the day. Also be aware if you're consuming lots of caffeine to try to make up for lack of sleep.

Don't dine late. Eating dinner late, especially if it's a big, heavy, or spicy meal, can mean you're still digesting when it's time for bed. In general, any food or snacks before bed should be on the lighter side. But also...

Don't go to bed hungry. If you've eaten early or are struggling to manage your blood sugars, try a small bedtime snack to stop cortisol spiking.

Restrict in-bed activity. To build a link in your mind between sleep and being in bed, it's best to only use your bed for sleep, with sex being the one exception.

Optimize your bedroom. A central component of sleep hygiene beyond just habits is your sleep environment. To fall asleep more easily, you want your bedroom to emanate tranquillity. While what makes a bedroom inviting can vary from one person to the next, these tips may help make it calm and free of disruptions:

- **Have a comfortable mattress and pillow.** Your sleeping surface is critical to comfort and pain-free sleep, so choose the best mattress and best pillow for your needs.

- **Use excellent bedding.** The sheets and blankets are the first thing you touch when you get into bed, so it's beneficial to make sure they match your needs and preferences.

- **Set a cool yet comfortable temperature.** Fine-tune your bedroom temperature to suit your preferences but err on the cooler side (around 18°C or 65°F).

- **Block out light.** Use heavy curtains or an eye mask to prevent light from interrupting your sleep.

- **Drown out noise.** Ear plugs can stop noise from keeping you awake; if you don't find them comfortable, you can try a white noise machine or even a fan to drown out bothersome sounds.

It sounds like a lot, but having a checklist to help you have an excellent night's sleep really does make a big change to our health and stress.

Do the right exercise

Doing the wrong exercise is as a detrimental for our body as doing no exercise.

That may sound like a bold claim, but one of the most common mistakes we see is when women do the wrong kind of exercise.

As women start to put weight on during perimenopause, they often panic and start running or doing high-intensity training. Bearing in mind that intense fatigue is a common symptom of perimenopause, they are often dragging themselves to do this exercise in the name of being healthy. It's not. It is also important to exercise at the right time of the day.

What do we mean by the right time of day?

Our stress hormone, cortisol, is supposed to peak in the morning.

This is the best time of day to exercise, especially if we are experiencing sleep issues or exhaustion. Working with our circadian rhythms helps the body regulate itself. Doing a hard workout in the evening means we start spiking our cortisol too late in the day, and this reduces our ability to switch into the parasympathetic nervous system response and keeps us wired. This in turn means we produce more insulin and store fat, which is usually the opposite of what we are trying to achieve.

Gentle exercise is OK in the evening. A sunset walk or a yoga class can be a wonderful way to wind down, but it is not the time for running or big workouts.

What is the right exercise? It depends on how you are feeling.

It is never a good idea to exercise if you are truly exhausted, but generally during perimenopause, we would recommend avoiding high-impact cardiovascular exercise like running and opt for low-impact cardiovascular exercise like cycling. And lifting weights.

Pretty much all the doctors and fitness professionals agree that working with weights is essential because weight bearing is one of the best ways to avoid osteoporosis, diminished bone density, and reduced muscle mass.

When you build muscle, you balance your blood sugars, reduce fat storage, balance your blood pressure, and maintain strong bones. Building muscle means lifting heavy things, but if you've never lifted before, start gently.

Find a weight you can lift to ten repetitions with ease. You then start to add weight until you're struggling to get to six repetitions.

If you are unsure, maybe you can book a few sessions with a personal trainer to help you find a routine that works for you, or, as a cheaper option, buy an online programme.

EMF exposure
What are EMFs?
EMFs, or electromagnetic fields, are invisible areas of energy or lines of force that emanate from matter. Our bodies have electric and magnetic fields that are associated with our nervous and muscular systems. The Earth also has a natural magnetic field, and there are electric fields in the atmosphere.

Usually when we refer to EMF exposure and health risks, we are talking about the electromagnetic fields that come from our electrical devices. This kind of EMF exposure comes from our phones, our cars, power lines, laptops, mobile phone towers, and Wi-Fi.

We are now very exposed to EMF in a way that no other generation has been exposed previously, and many people are starting to be concerned about the effect on their health.

Are EMFs dangerous?
Most of us live in a home with our Wi-Fi on 24/7, a smart meter attached to the outside of our living room wall, and our iPhone by our head as we sleep. Our children play with our mobile phones or use electronics to learn and play. This EMF-infused technology has become a way of life for many of us.

We need to be careful. There is a growing body of scientific evidence showing that too much EMF exposure can be harmful to our health. In fact, in 2011 the World Health Organization classified EMFs as "possibly carcinogenic to humans" after EMF radiation was linked to a specific type of brain cancer.[6]

Here are some EMF exposure symptoms to look out for:

- chronic headaches

- excessive fatigue

- feeling of stress or being "wired"

- trouble sleeping soundly through the night

- tingling, burning, or prickling skin sensations

- a buzzing or static feeling in brain

- ringing ears

- unexplained rashes or hives

- body pain

- weakened immunity

- hormonal imbalances that won't respond to treatment.

How to reduce EMF exposure
Caution with mobile phones
Did you know that every phone comes with a warning about keeping the phone too close to your body? In fact, the iPhone manual states that users should keep the phone ten millimetres away from their ear. Either use the speaker function or wired headphones.

Easy on the home Wi-Fi
A great practice is to turn off your Wi-Fi router before you go to bed.

Be smart about your smart meter
A hidden source of EMFs in your home could come from your smart meter. This meter is an electronic device that records electric energy consumption. Many people report health problems after being in proximity to smart meters, so be sure your home is safe.

Get into nature
Spending time in nature can act as a balm for our busy brains. Research has shown that interacting with nature has cognitive benefits. Other studies have found that being exposed to natural environments improves working memory, cognition, and attention control.[7]

The diversity of bacteria and fungi in nature is strengthening for our immune response and supports our gut microbiome more effectively than taking probiotics in supplement form.

Research suggests that even just the view of a forest from a hospital room helps boost mood, and as little as 20 minutes spent in nature could significantly reduce your levels of cortisol.[8] It feels like a no-brainer if we are trying to reduce stress!

Deal with your emotional issues

Emotions are major stressors if we haven't learned tools to navigate them.

Developing emotional resilience is not something that happens naturally. It is something that must be learned and practised. Like a muscle, we need to keep developing it with repeated exercise. This then needs to be followed by self-reflection.

Many behaviours such as caretaking, people pleasing, having no boundaries, and lying to ourselves and others are the result of conditioning and a deep-seated fear of rejection and being unloved and alone. But neither the behaviours nor fears serve us, and instead they create a deep lack of self-love and a requirement for external validation and acceptance, which leads to anxiety, depression, and an inability to say no.

On a very primal level, our instincts are always trying to keep us safe. In the prehistoric era, we learned to listen to our guts because they would save us from attack: we could run away or get eaten. Today we are no longer running from wild animals, but we can experience the same response when we are reacting to an emotion.

Research suggests that suppressing emotions is associated with high rates of heart disease, as well as autoimmune disorders, ulcers, IBS, and gastrointestinal health complications. When we suppress emotions, whether anger, sadness, grief, or frustration, the act of pushing those feelings aside leads to physical stress on the body.

Studies show that holding in feelings has a correlation with high cortisol – the hormone released in response to stress – and that cortisol leads to lower immunity and toxic thinking patterns. Over time, untreated or unrecognized stress can lead to an increased risk of diabetes, aggression, anxiety, and depression.

In other words, deciding to bury your feelings, ignore them, internalize them, pretend they didn't happen, or convince yourself that there is no need to deal with them can literally make you sick from the stress.

The official term for getting unwell because of our emotions or the stress on our nervous system is psychoneuroimmunology and psychoneuroendocrinology – the study of how our psychology affects our nervous system and immune system or hormones.

We call it the "emotion–health connection".

And the truth is that we cannot be truly well until we have cleared our baggage. It's never too late, and menopause is the perfect time to do this work as our hormones and tolerance change, and we have that lack of tolerance developing that makes it easier to put in boundaries.

But this isn't easy to do by ourselves.

We are passionate about how this work can change lives. We've spent 25 years learning these tools and we adore supporting people to do this work. We have also trained multiple dozens of coaches and practitioners to be able to support clients to go through emotional transformation. There are many ways to get started.

Try an online course like our Reclaim Your Life programme, do some ongoing one-to-one work with a coach, or, if you want to dive into an immersive experience, attend an emotional development retreat. We have put links to these options in Chapter 16 on next steps and resources.

Menopause is a time of shedding the old and transitioning into a new phase of life. It's the perfect time to get rid of your baggage and make the changes so that you can be who you choose to be as you enter your third age.

Structural stressors

Joint pains, jaw problems, gut issues, and backache all add masses of stress to the body, and they really don't have to.

We strongly recommend finding a local kinesiologist or body worker who can help you align the underlying structure of your body. If that would cost too much, seek out training colleges looking for case studies to work with their students. But don't suffer in silence.

Summary

Although progressive thought leaders in the scientific community believe that many of these factors are involved with inflammation and chronic illness, the fact that there isn't a direct and clear-cut approach to reducing the impact of this list means that it is hard for doctors to make recommendations. The lifestyle changes feel too broad and vague and there is no medication that will solve any of these issues.

Supporting people to make the necessary lifestyle changes and provide education around them takes time, and we know that time is a resource that doctors generally don't have available. But to create lasting whole-health solutions, it is important to have awareness of the impact of these factors and make changes step by step.

TAKE-HOME MESSAGE

There are a lot of areas that need addressing for us to reduce the impact of stress on our body. We can't do it all overnight. Step by step is the way to go here, making one embedded change at a time.

A lot of these changes only require us to bring awareness to what's needed and tweak it. Many of them don't cost anything and can be implemented straight away.

If you do one thing on the list every day, in a few months you will have reduced the impact of stressors substantially on your body and freed up bandwidth.

— CHAPTER 12 —

Hormone replacement therapy (HRT)

To use HRT or not to use HRT? That is the question!

The decision about whether to take hormone replacement therapy or not is a truly individual one. What is right for some isn't right for all.

We are often asked our opinion on whether HRT is a good idea, and we always answer that it depends how much your symptoms are affecting your life. Menopause has such a broad spectrum of experience. Many women still sail through with only the occasional hot flush. Others cannot function and can barely get out of bed.

Our recommendation is to do the research, get all the information, and follow the path that feels right for you.

It's important to know that the decision is a double-edged sword. There are risks associated with taking HRT and there are risks associated with not taking HRT. Menopausal women really are stuck between a rock and a hard place in this regard.

However, there are options that have far fewer associated risks, and we are passionate about educating women on these options so they can make some clearly informed decisions.

The risks associated with HRT are explained throughout this chapter but, importantly, the risks associated with *not* taking HRT include:

- deteriorating skin health

- decreased bone health and increased risk of osteoporosis

- increased risk of heart disease

- vaginal atrophy

- poor memory/memory loss

- increased absenteeism at work.

Research shows that if you choose to take HRT, there is a time limit. Benefits are not seen if you wait longer than five years post-menopause to start taking it.

The difficulty in trying to find out information online is that most of the articles that talk about HRT and the risks associated with it aren't clarifying *which* HRT they are talking about.

We would argue that the natural HRT options are significantly different to the synthetic versions, but these articles are unclear and are most probably talking about synthetic versions as these are more widely available and have been used more commonly historically. As such, both options must be talked about as entirely separate entities, and as far as we can tell, this isn't happening.

Let's explore what these different options are. There are five types of hormone replacement available:

- synthetic hormone replacement therapy

- herbal supplements that support hormone production

- low-dose bioidentical hormone replacement therapy

- body-identical hormone replacement therapy

- compounded bioidentical hormone replacement therapy.

Synthetic hormone replacement therapy

The range of synthetic HRT products is staggering. They come in all different forms and have a variety of names, including:

- Mirena/Kyleena/Skyla coils

- combination pills (except for Bijuve which is bodyidentical)

- progesterone-only pills (except for Utrogestan, Geprentix and Cycolgest, which are body-identical)

- combination patches

- oestrogen-only patches (except for Estradot, which is body-identical)

- pessaries

- oestrogen gel.

The synthetic oestrogen and progesterone used in HRT and contraceptives come with serious side effects. These side effects are commonly discussed in the media.

According to a major study published in 2002, the risks of taking these medications – such as elevated risk of stroke, thrombosis, heart attacks, and pulmonary embolism – far exceeded the benefits of taking them.[1] Recent research, however, has suggested that there are different ways of managing risks for individual patients, and that the benefits outweigh the risks in women under the age of 60 and where there are no other contraindications present.[2]

We are not so sure, because not only do the synthetics often cause symptoms, but they can also stop our body from making its own progesterone, which is not good for our health. Evidence shows that combined hormonal contraceptives reduce the levels of oestrogen and progesterone in fertile women.[3]

Many types of combination pill or synthetic hormone patch are widely used as HRT when women are in perimenopause. There are two major issues with this: the progesterone used in these medications isn't progesterone, which we are about to explore, and the use of these medications leads to oestrogen dominance.

As we already know, perimenopause is characterized by progesterone dropping while oestrogen fluctuates, which already causes oestrogen dominance. By loading a body already saturated with oestrogen with more oestrogen, we see women struggling with many symptoms such as weight gain, insulin resistance, exhaustion, mood swings, and memory issues.

Research shows that other issues such as breast cancer and strokes are also linked to excess oestrogen. The picture we looked at in Part One is that most women are already in oestrogen dominance due to xeno-oestrogens and poor diet, so we are taking women who are naturally in a place of oestrogen dominance, exacerbated by xeno-oestrogens, and loading them up with massive doses of synthetic oestrogen and no proper progesterone to stop the fallout.

Does that make sense? No, we don't think so either.

We have got to a point where these medications are used for a broad spectrum of conditions as opposed to just being for birth control or HRT.

The medical reliance on these medications rests on the delusion that synthetic hormonal contraception is a substitute for real human hormones. It is not a substitute. The drugs in the pill, patch, or implant are not hormones, and it is important to remember that pill bleeds are not periods.

On top of this, many women are told to have certain products – for example, the Mirena coil – because GP surgeries can be financially incentivized to prescribe them. It is common to hear stories of women being refused when they ask to have them removed. Often, these decisions are not being made about women's health but economics. If that seems like too harsh an evaluation, it might be fairer to say that the decision cannot possibly be unbiased when financial incentivization is a carrot being dangled in front of prescribing practitioners.

What do we mean exactly when we say that the synthetic hormones aren't really hormones? Let's look at them one by one.

Oestrogen

Oestrogen is a generic term. It can be used to refer to anything oestrogenic such as oestradiol, ethinylestradiol in the pill, and xeno-oestrogens from the environment.

Synthetic oestrogen is like the oestrogen the body makes but isn't identical to it, and synthetic oestrogens are usually stronger than human oestrogens.

These synthetics can cause the liver and bowel to work harder to metabolize them and may cause a build-up in the body, which contributes to the oestrogen overloads we are seeing throughout society and causes the side effects of oestrogen dominance.

Combined with the fact that so many women are on synthetic oestrogens that are excreted out that we now have high levels of xeno-oestrogen in our water supply and in the food chain, this means that xeno-oestrogen levels in humans are elevating.

Bioidentical oestrogen isn't as strong and mimics more closely the hormone we make, which means it is easier to metabolize.

It is interesting to note that in HRT medications, oestrogen in the form of oestradiol is only used when post-menopausal women need oestriol. Many women find a combination of both types of oestrogen more beneficial than the overstimulating effects of oestradiol alone.

Is a synthetic option ever a good idea? Well, surprisingly, yes.

For women who are struggling with vaginal dryness, the oestrogen pessaries are incredibly helpful, and many women prefer to have the oestrogen gel pump because they don't like the idea of a patch. The trick is to be aware of what oestrogen dominance symptoms are – such as tender breasts and headaches – so you know if you have too much. In this instance, speak to your GP about reducing the dose.

Progesterone

To quote Q in the James Bond movies, "Pay attention, 007." This is probably the most important information in this book and the part we have been building up to.

The chemicals in any synthetic HRT, contraceptive pill, patch, implant, hormonal coil, or the mini pill *are not progesterone*. They are chemical compounds referred to as "progestins". They are called drospirenone, levonorgestrel, or medroxyprogesterone, and as you can see in the diagrams below, they look different to progesterone.

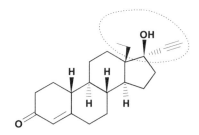

DIAGRAM 23 – THE CHEMICAL STRUCTURE OF SYNTHETIC PROGESTIN

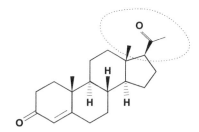

DIAGRAM 24 – THE CHEMICAL STRUCTURE OF NATURAL PROGESTERONE

The images shows the chemical difference between levonorgestrel, which is the progestin used in many oral contraceptives, implants, the Mirena coil, and the morning-after pill, and natural progesterone.

Chemically, these are totally different. Levonorgestrel is more similar to testosterone than it is to progesterone (which is problematic because, as we know, progesterone is a calming hormone whereas testosterone is an exciter hormone).

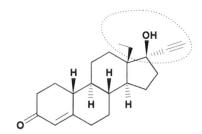

DIAGRAM 23 – THE CHEMICAL STRUCTURE OF SYNTHETIC PROGESTIN

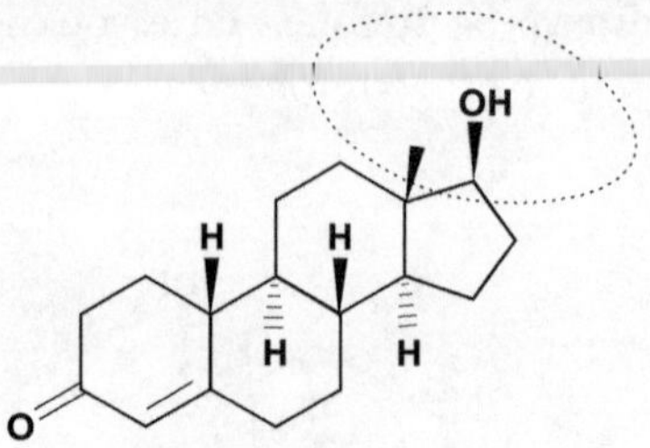

DIAGRAM 25 – THE CHEMICAL STRUCTURE OF TESTOSTERONE

This is important because of how they affect the body.
Progesterone:

- is beneficial for cardiovascular health

- stimulates hair growth

- calms mood and promotes sleep

- prevents breast cancer

- is anti-inflammatory.

Progestin:

- increases the risk of fatal blood clots

- can cause hair loss (due to its similarity to testosterone)

- may cause anxiety and depression

- increases the risk of breast cancer.

Women need progesterone to support adrenal function. Remember, when we are too stressed, we prioritize producing cortisol over progesterone. We need that calming action when we are stressed a lot more than we need more "upregulating" hormones.

One of the "big picture" issues with these hormones is that due to the pregnenolone steal, the fact that during menopause our adrenal glands take over making progesterone, and the fact that being oestrogen dominant is a large "stressor", the exposure to the fake progesterone stops our body's ability to make any progesterone at all. Therefore, women who are desperately in need of progesterone become more and more depleted in progesterone and unable to make it.

We cannot stress this highly enough. If women are taking a synthetic progesterone, they are not getting any benefits from that progesterone – in fact, it could be causing damage to their overall health and wellbeing.

— 172 —

Women are commonly told by the GP that the progesterone in the hormonal coil provides localized progesterone. That isn't true. According to the FDA website, the progesterone still shows in blood plasma; there's just less of it than with the pill.[4]

This device is offered to millions and millions of women and heralded as the answer to all their hormone issues, not just menopause. Women have been lulled into a belief that not bleeding is convenient, and this device is beneficial. It isn't. It's masking the underlying issues but can be contributing to far more serious issues. The authors Lara Briden and Nicole Jardim (www. nicolejardim.com, www.larabriden.com) have both covered this topic extensively, and it is important information for all women to know.

In the 2000s, the popularity of HRT dropped dramatically after the World Health Institute published a study showing post-menopausal women taking combination (oestrogen and progesterone) hormone therapy had an increased risk for breast cancer, heart disease, stroke, blood clots, and urinary incontinence.[5] This study was started in 1991 as a proposed 15-year study. Menopausal women with a uterus were randomized to take a placebo or PremPro®, a combination of Premarin® – an adapted horse oestrogen (premarin is a contraction of "pregnant mares' urine") and medroxyprogesterone, a synthetic version of progesterone.

In 2002, the study was stopped early due to a statistical increase in breast cancer and stroke, and no apparent benefit for reducing cardiovascular risk. This sent shockwaves around the world, and women everywhere pulled away from using HRT out of fear of developing breast cancer. HRT saw a drop of 8 per cent in some countries and a 68 per cent reduction in others.

The limitation of this study was the type of oestrogen and progestin used. Premarin contains ten different oestrogens but almost no oestradiol, the most powerful of the body's oestrogens. Taken as an oestrogen pill, it is absorbed in the intestine, with a "first pass" through the liver, increasing production of many clotting factors. This explains the increased incidence of stroke in the study. Interestingly, transdermal oestrogen via gel, spray, or patch does not stimulate these clotting factors.

Medroxyprogesterone was used as the progestin. Recent data suggests that medroxyprogesterone in breast tissue may alter hormone receptors adjacent to the oestrogen receptors, increasing the risks of oestrogen-stimulated cancers.

When it comes to understanding the relationship between breast cancer, sex hormone receptors, and HRT, it is important to consider the power of natural progesterone over synthetic progestin alternatives and unopposed oestrogen. The emergence of breast cancer often coincides with the peri-menopause, when women are naturally oestrogen dominant. Supporting and promoting natural progesterone production in perimenopause could protect against breast cancer.

The use of synthetic progestins isn't just a problem with HRT.

Many, many women are offered the synthetic hormones at a young age. We believe the use of the pill is overprescribed for conditions it was never designed to treat. Issues such as PCOS, endometriosis, adenomyosis, PMDD, fibroids, amenorrhea, and dysmenorrhea have their roots in oestrogen dominance, insulin resistance, and inflammation. Treating these disorders with medications that contribute to furthering oestrogen dominance, inhibiting natural progesterone production, and adding to inflammation and insulin resistance is insanity.

The use of these medications for conditions arising from oestrogen dominance can lead to serious health issues such as strokes and deep vein thrombosis, and complicate underlying oestrogen dominance, which has health ramifications for women, often for the rest of their lives.

It is surprisingly common for women to never get their cycle back because of the damage caused by these drugs due to issues such as "post-pill PCOS" or pituitary gland failure, but we have never, ever heard of a woman being warned of these side effects by a doctor so that she could make an informed choice.

When these medications don't work – which they commonly do not – women are often offered a hysterectomy or other surgical interventions.

Artificial hormones or surgery aren't the answer – natural progesterone, better diet, and reduced stress are more likely to be.

The piece of the puzzle that is perplexing is that the medical model will offer synthetic progesterone for these conditions, but when our clients ask for natural progesterone, they are told that "this isn't how we work with these conditions". We believe this needs a radical review.

However, saying all that, some women get on well with synthetic hormones and feel like they have solved all the problems menopause brought with it. We celebrate the women who feel great on them, but for long-term health we would also encourage them to look at less toxic versions. We are, however, more interested in getting the message out that many, many women cannot tolerate synthetic HRT and are left without support or guidance. These are the women we want to reach, to show them that there are other options and they aren't alone!

Herbal supplements that support hormone production

Herbs have been used to reduce menopause symptoms since the dawn of time and there are far too many to quote here. Every practitioner will have herbs that they favour, and it seems like each week something else is being promoted.

Traditionally, herbs like dong quai, black cohosh, and red clover are commonly taken, and although many women find them very beneficial, those having a challenging menopause often need something with more "oomph".

The herbs we tend to work with have a direct interaction with our hormones and support the body to produce more of what we need.

Chaste tree (*Vitex agnus-castus*) is a natural progesterone booster. It can be game-changing during early perimenopause.

Ashwagandha promotes testosterone production and is great for tiredness and apathy.

Gelatinized maca root is *phenomenal* for hot flushes. This has high levels of phyto-oestrogens – 3 teaspoons daily for three weeks can stop hot flushes in their tracks.

Soy is another great oestrogen booster. Taken in the form of capsules, shakes, or eaten as tofu or soy mince, the only time we recommend soy is when women are deeply into the menopause transition and starting to miss bleeds. Soy is a powerful phyto-oestrogen and not helpful if you are in the oestrogen dominance phase.

Evening primrose oil is another commonly used phyto-oestrogen. As with the others, we recommend using this later in your transition, so you don't contribute to oestrogen dominance.

Please speak with a practitioner before using herbs, and if you've had any hormone-related cancers or autoimmune conditions, it is imperative you check with your doctor. While these are totally natural, they are powerful and must not be underestimated.

One current craze involves seed cycling. Seed cycling involves eating flax, pumpkin, sesame, and sunflower seeds at different times of your menstrual cycle. The practice is claimed to balance hormones, and ease symptoms of menopause. However, evidence to support these claims is either lacking or weak. We aren't fans of seed cycling because seeds can be highly sensitizing to people with intestinal permeability or IBS, and seeds contain high levels of omega 6, which is inflammatory. But some women swear by it, and as with everything we talk about, whatever gets you through this challenging time must be applauded!

Low-dose bioidentical hormone replacement therapy

Low-dose bioidentical HRT is available in the form of progesterone creams, oestriol creams, DHEA (dehydroepiandrosterone), and pregnenolone (not testosterone), and these were readily available in the UK through practitioners like kinesiologists. This was until spring 2023 when we discovered that suppliers were no longer able to import these helpful products.

Low-dose bioidentical hormones were life-changing for women struggling with being "tired but wired" and having adrenal fallouts during their early perimenopause, along with the associated symptoms of insomnia and brain fog. We are devastated that these have been removed from circulation.

Body-identical hormone replacement therapy

Body-identical hormones are the same compounds as bioidentical hormones, but they are NHS-regulated products. The body-identical hormones available from the GP are fantastic.

These are essentially made from yams, like the bioidentical hormones, but they are stronger than the low-dose bioidentical options.

The body-identical oestrogen is called Estradot and this comes in a patch form.

The body-identical progesterone is called Utrogestan in the UK and Europe, and Prometrium in the USA and Australia. Some GPs issue this without a problem, others don't, and many haven't heard about it, but women are within their rights to be put on this more natural form of HRT.

The downsides to Utrogestan are that it contains peanut and soy, and women who have allergies or intolerances to these ingredients won't be able to take this product. It is in capsule form, and women with a history of gut issues may struggle to absorb the progesterone. There is a vaginal pessary version, but many women complain as they create an extremely sticky and claggy residue, and it can feel a bit like your vagina has been filled with glue (as Claire likes to call it, "clag vag"). It's not a pleasant experience and can create quite a lot of vaginal soreness. Another issue with Utrogestan is that the micronized progesterone can cause a bit of intermittent spotting, and many women aren't happy with this experience.

Other troubleshooting tips

We often see women being given Utrogestan, but due to a lack of understanding or training on the part of the GP, the prescription can be inappropriate. Utrogestan was originally created as a fertility drug, meaning it was given to women who were in their fertile years and who still had a cycle without the drop-off in progesterone we see in perimenopause. Because of this, Utrogestan is supposed to support the cycle with progesterone coming in at ovulation (day 14) and reducing on the day before a bleed (day 27). Utrogestan is therefore commonly given from days 14 to 28 only. This is ideal for women with a regular cycle who have conditions such as PMDD, but it is not useful at all for a perimenopausal woman who doesn't have enough progesterone to carry her through the rest of the cycle. Progesterone is always present in our cycle; it just peaks on days 14–28.

If a woman has had some menstrual irregularities, she often won't even know when day 14 or 25 is supposed to be in her cycle!

We also see women being given it for days 1–25 and then a few days' break. Again, this is irrelevant if she has no cycle.

It is important to remember that progesterone does so much more than just thicken our endometrial lining. It helps our mood and sleep, regulates stress hormones, assists in weight control and appetite control, and reduces inflammation. We need that every day!

Women are also sometimes not given enough progesterone. If a woman has had a history of trauma, major ill health, chronic fatigue, high stress, or autoimmune issues, one capsule of 100mg might not be enough. The phenomenal research at the Centre for Menstrual Cycle and Ovulation Research (CeMCOR) at the University of British Columbia in Canada highlighted the benefit of high-dose progesterone therapy.[6] Although GPs can't support a dose that is over the licensed allowance, they can support a dose that goes up to the licensed allowance. This is 200mg and the in-packet guidance refers to "1 or 2" capsules (one capsule is 100mg).

Our recommendation is that if you've been taking one tablet and you haven't noticed any great change, go back to your doctor and ask them to support trialling an increased dose.

Claire found a doctor who supported a high-dose trial. She needed 400mg for a year which reduced to 300mg for six months before dropping to 200mg, which has been her standard dose for three years. With her history of trauma and chronic fatigue, this isn't surprising as there was a huge history of progesterone deficiency. Hers is a specific case, and we don't advocate this as a common approach; we are using it here to illustrate that 200mg isn't a huge dose, just the top end of the licensed allowance.

The only reported side effects are increased drowsiness (which can be a godsend for menopausal women with insomnia) and the uterus lining thickening too much – which a scan will show.

Research shows that progesterone is incredibly important in menopause and that it is progesterone that supports bone density as opposed to oestrogen.[7] It's time for the NHS to wake up to this.

GPs usually only prescribe oestrogen and progesterone but not testosterone, DHEA, or pregnenolone, which is often not a full solution for women. Some doctors will work with testosterone, but again it's a lottery. This is something that is being campaigned about by the menopause celebrities, and a victory would be a huge leap forward.

As an example of low-dose bioidenticals versus standard dose of body-identicals – the bioidentical progesterone starts at 4mg per drop. Utrogestan is 100mg. This means women can be supported with bioidenticals much earlier on in the perimenopause transition.

We are passionate about supporting women to be able to ask their GP for body-identical hormones if it is medically appropriate. It is common, however, for women to be refused this option or be told they need to see specialists for a prescription, which will take a year or so, or that the NHS doesn't offer it. This is not true. Push back.

On our website, we have an open letter to GPs to support our clients in requesting this course of medication. This link is included in the resources in Chapter 16.

Women shouldn't have to work so hard to get the support they need at a time when they feel scared, confused, and vulnerable, but we do.

Ask the questions. Remember, GPs are often not trained in menopause, many don't know what options are available, and you may find you give them useful information. Trust what you have learned, and don't allow anyone to medically gaslight you or put you down.

We hear these stories daily and it is heart-breaking.

There are also stories of great GPs who are supportive and understand, but as we've said before, it's a lottery, and your best approach is to go in with your knowledge and request what you want. It is your right if there is no *medical* reason that you can't.

There are also exciting developments in the field of autoimmune disease with regard to progesterone.

One study found women with rheumatoid arthritis exhibited significantly lower progesterone levels during the luteal phase of the menstrual cycle compared to the control group, suggesting its protective role in autoimmune conditions.[8]

Compounded bioidentical hormone replacement therapy

For women who are having a challenging menopause, who might have a history of gut issues, who can't tolerate Utrogestan, or who have progesterone sensitivity, there is another option.

This option is not regulated or advocated by the NHS – in fact, many doctors actively dissuade women from this pathway. However, for the women who have nowhere left to turn, it is a route that can literally give them back their quality of life.

There are many excellent specialist doctors who work with high-dose bioidentical hormones. These doctors also offer testosterone, DHEA, and pregnenolone as well as progesterone and oestrogen. They use blood tests to ascertain what bespoke blend of hormones is needed and these are then created in laboratories specifically for the individual. These solutions are very effective but very expensive (hundreds of pounds a month in some cases) and therefore not readily accessible to many women. As mentioned, they are also unregulated, so the NHS argument is that you don't know what you are getting. Speaking from personal experience, this option changed Claire's life, and she wouldn't have been able to get back to work or off prescription sleep medication without it.

Big picture review

In very early perimenopause (from late 30s), women start to notice tiny signs that are often ignored or attributed to stress. Doctors often overlook these signs. These can include weight gain, drop in confidence in everyday things like driving, forgetfulness (putting their keys in the fridge), an increase in urinating, increased food intolerance, low mood, increased anxiety, the feeling of "spinning too many plates", insomnia, being snappy, low libido, and fatigue. Sometimes this is when women are diagnosed with thyroid issues as more pressure is put on the thyroid; this is often a victim of these hormonal changes. Women are also often prescribed antidepressants and beta blockers at this time.

These are key indicators that progesterone is starting to drop. Working on reducing oestrogen dominance using lifestyle changes, supplements like DIM (diindolylmethan), NAC (N-acetyl-L-cysteine), and calcium D-glucarate, and herbs such as chaste tree can be life-changing. In other cases, finding a practitioner who works with low-dose bioidentical hormones can help. Sometimes women respond to progesterone, but often in early perimeno-pause they respond more to pregnenolone, meaning their body can convert that pregnenolone to the progesterone they need with this low-dose support and they don't need the big doses yet.

What about high-dose oestrogen therapy?

There is a huge culture of administering high doses of oestrogen. This is advocated by a few celebrity doctors but has gained traction among a lot of GPs.

The science behind this approach is scant, and in 2023 a large-scale investigation was initiated as thousands of women have been injured and harmed with this trend. This has been widely reported in the media, with amounts being prescribed above of licensed levels.[9]

We do not advocate it. If anything, we hope the message that we have conveyed is that we see a lack of progesterone as a huge issue and oestrogen dominance as a major culprit. Please take heed: our clinics have seen the fallout and the damage caused to dozens and dozens of women who have been issued high-dose oestrogen therapy.

Hormones should never be issued at a high dose for any length of time without regular blood tests and careful monitoring. This must not become a standard approach for all women. High doses of oestrogen dramatically increase the chances of stroke, embolism, cancer, and other issues such as migraines, digestive issues, depression, insomnia, and weight gain.

When is it time to come off HRT?

The answer, again, is that it is up to the individual.

Some women feel so great on HRT that they don't intend to come off it at all. Although this isn't recommended with synthetic hormones, there is much less risk associated with body-identical hormones. Other women want to come off HRT as soon as they can.

With all these decisions, it is imperative that you create a plan with your doctor.

What we do want to highlight, however, is that women are often unaware that they will have a hormone withdrawal when they come off HRT. It is referred to as a "second menopause". Our understanding, however, is that if you have fully transitioned through menopause and your hormones have stabilized, then you will only be dealing with the hormonal withdrawal from coming off HRT, instead of dealing with both the massive hormone roller-coaster of the menopause transition and a hormone withdrawal.

It's important to think through all these issues before deciding so that you feel comfortable with your choices.

— CHAPTER 13 —

What is the best diet during menopause?

One of the most common questions we are asked is "What is a healthy diet?" and our answer is always "What are you trying to achieve?" Ultimately, it depends on what is happening with your health profile and what your goals are, but there are some basics that we all need to adhere to if we want those strong foundations of health.

Sadly, these basics are hugely overlooked and undertaught. Many of the symptoms we see in clinic could be avoided with just a little bit of education about how to eat in a way that supports our body.

The most important aspect of learning how to eat healthily is understanding the macronutrients.

Understanding macronutrients

There are three macronutrients: protein, fats, and carbohydrates. They are called macronutrients because we need a lot of them in our diet. All our food is made up of the macronutrients.

What is protein?

Proteins are large molecules made up of amino acids. Protein and amino acids are the building blocks for life, and they play many critical roles in the body.

We will be talking about two types of protein: the macronutrient protein that we eat (such as meat, eggs, tofu, and fish) and the proteins we make in the body to carry out specific functions. They are interwoven because the protein we eat breaks down into amino acids, which we then use to make our internal proteins, essential for vital functions,

Unless we eat protein, our body literally doesn't function properly.

Protein also boosts your metabolism every time you eat it, and if you remember from Chapter 4, the protein leverage hypothesis states that mammals are in a heightened state of anxiety until they consume enough protein. That shows how important it is.

Sadly, many diets are depleted in protein, and this causes many issues with health.

The proteins we make in our body ensure we function properly. Proteins play a role in nearly every biological process. Our cells cannot function without them, and they are required for structure, strength, and repair.

Examples of proteins that have a bodily function are:

- structural proteins such as collagen or keratin

- hormones such as insulin

- carriers, such as haemoglobin in our red blood cells which carry oxygen in the bloodstream

- enzymes, such as the ones made in our stomach and pancreas to digest our food.

What are fats?

Regardless of what the low-fat movement said in the 1980s, fat is essential for health. The knock-on effect of the low-fat trend is that many people are still scared of having fat in their diet as they believe it is either going to be detrimental to their health or make them put on weight.

We want to make this very clear. Natural fat from whole foods does not make you fat. In fact, it helps regulate our hormones and can even aid with weight loss.

Fat has multiple essential functions in the body:

- It functions as an energy reserve, meaning we can break it down and use it as fuel.

- It is how we absorb fat-soluble vitamins like vitamins A, D, E, and K.

- It keeps hair and skin healthy.

- It insulates the body and protects organs.

- As we explored in Chapter 6, it is part of the production process for oestrogen, progesterone, and testosterone (yes, fat makes hormones!).

- It balances blood sugars.

- It helps fight infection.

- It reduces inflammation.

- And the fat we eat is what makes our food taste good and helps with satisfaction.

Fats in our diet come in different forms. To understand these fully, we need to study organic chemistry and dive deeply into hydrogen bonds and long-chain fatty acids, which can be tough going. There are other books that do that better than we could, so instead we will give you an overview.

Saturated fats

Until very recently, saturated fats were considered "bad fats". The data linking dietary fat with heart disease is weak at best and corrupt at worst. The exception to this is the data we have on hydrogenated fats, which are also called trans fats. It was considered that because fat in the form of cholesterol is found in the arteries of people with cardiovascular disease, it *must* be fat in the diet causing this. But as we've already explored, a build-up of cholesterol is due to inflammation, and this is more likely to be because of stress and eating food we are intolerant to. In fact, in some studies, the people involved were eating burgers (and many of them smoked), but when they were shown to have elevated cholesterol, it was assumed that it was the meat that caused the issue, not the bun, the processed cheese, the fries, or the cigarettes.

This data could not have been more wrong. In fact, we know that there is very little evidence of saturated fats being bad at all, and there is now more evidence that eating a diet with regular consumption of saturated fat is in line with our evolution and essential for health. The benefits of eating saturated fat include cardiovascular and brain health.

Saturated fats are the simplest fatty acids and are often hard at room temperature.

There are different types of saturated fats, and they are classified depending on how long the chain of fatty acids is:

- **Short-chain fatty acids** are found in meat and dairy products such as butter, lard, suet, crackling, and bacon fat.

- **Medium-chain fatty acids** (also called medium-chain triglycerides) are found in a processed form of coconut oil.

- **Long-chain fatty acids** are solid at body temperature and make up cell membranes. Examples are beef, lamb, pork, cheese, and coconut oil.

Saturated fats are essential for good health. We have evolved to be able to eat them abundantly, and as we explored in Chapter 11, when we eat saturated fats, the stearic acid sends signals to our body that it is safe to be in a fat-burning state as opposed to a fat-storage state, which is part of the mechanism that reduces inflammation.

Monounsaturated fats

Monounsaturated fats (or MUFAs) are liquid at room temperature and begin to solidify when refrigerated. The most common monounsaturated fatty acid is oleic acid, which is found in foods such as olive oil, avocados, olives, and nuts.

Monounsaturated fats are considered healthy fats, offering a number of benefits. They:

- protect against heart disease and metabolic syndrome
- are anti-inflammatory
- benefit heart arrhythmia
- improve insulin sensitivity
- support weight loss
- improve mood
- strengthen bones.

Polyunsaturated fats

Polyunsaturated fats (or PUFAs) tend to be vegetable oils or seed oils. They are currently coming into the spotlight as being one of the primary causes of dietary inflammation and insulin resistance (along with wheat and sugar).

The main offenders are coined the "hateful eight" and include oils made from rapeseed, cottonseed, corn, grapeseed, rice bran, soy, sunflower, and safflower. These can be hiding in plain sight under the vague phrase "vegetable oil".

They are essentially industrial lubricants that are marketed to sound healthy, and they are cheap, which means that they are present in most ultra-processed food. The oils become rancid during the process of being chemically altered, and this is also a trigger for inflammation.

A diet high in PUFAs can lead to non-alcohol-induced liver disease, cardiovascular disease, and an increase in hunger. These oils really are toxic sludge that are contributing to major inflammation and disease in humans, and have no place in a healthy diet.

The only naturally occurring beneficial polyunsaturated fats are omega 3 oils from algae or fish, which are also called essential fatty acids (EFAs). They are called essential fatty acids because they are essential in our diet, and we can't manufacture them. They are not called "probably-a-good-idea fatty acids" or "if-I-can-be-bothered-to-include-them fatty acids". They are essential for good health.

Many people buy supplements containing omega 3, 6, and 9, but omega 6 and 9 are another form of vegetable or seed oil, and too much of them can cause inflammation. We must ensure we are taking omega 3 on its own.

Omega 3 is anti-inflammatory, and it has also been shown to prevent heart disease and stroke, and help control some autoimmune conditions.

However, if you want to rely on getting your omega 3 from eating fish, it is important to know that farmed fish is fed food which is full of the wrong kind of fats, and the fish itself can become too high in omega 6. Opting for wild fish is the best option.

Hydrogenated or trans fats

Trans fats are the worst kind of fats to eat. They are created as part of an industrial process that involves hydrogenation, where the chemical structure of fatty acid chains is changed and turned from a liquid fat into a solid or a semi-solid fat, making them more stable for longer shelf lives. The fats are then unnaturally saturated and harden at body temperature. Trans fats create a build-up of fatty material in the arteries and contribute to systemic inflammation when they are ingested.

Examples of hydrogenated trans fats include fast food, ultra-processed foods, margarine, fried foods, biscuits, doughnuts, and commercially made cakes and pies.

An excess of trans fats in your diet contributes to unhealthy cholesterol, heart disease, obesity, diabetes, insulin resistance, and metabolic syndrome.

Carbohydrates

Carbohydrates are a contentious subject these days. Some schools of thought say that carbohydrates are essential for health while others say they are not essential and increase your risk of developing many conditions.

People are often confused about what carbohydrates are. They are the sugars, starches, and fibres found in:

- dairy products
- fruits
- vegetables
- grains
- legumes
- sugary foods and confectionary.

Carbohydrates are the easiest way our body can make energy. They support brain function, muscle protection, and regulation of the central nervous system. They are also beneficial for the thyroid and hormone regulation.

Although there is no doubt that they are beneficial in a healthy diet, humans the world over have become carbohydrate addicts.

It is common for people to say that they "don't eat sugar" but their diet is full of fruit, grains, and root vegetables. While these are nutrient rich, it is important to remember that once the carbohydrates are broken down in the bowel, they are just sugar.

Diets full of vegetables, porridge, granola, toast, rice, pasta, potatoes or sweet potatoes, fruit, and quinoa all sound healthy, but when these are consumed without being balanced with protein and fats, we overload our bodies with carbohydrates and therefore cause blood sugar destabilization.

Carbohydrates are classified as either simple or complex.

Simple carbohydrates

These are sugars such as glucose, sucrose, fructose, and lactose. They are found in foods such as raw sugar, cane sugar, sweets, fruit juices, vegetable juices, fizzy drinks, and corn syrup. They don't yield any vitamins or minerals and provide "empty calories". These simple carbohydrates are absorbed very quickly, meaning they cause quick blood sugar spikes which then lead to blood sugar destabilization.

Complex carbohydrates

Complex carbohydrates are made up of sugar molecules strung together in long chains. They take longer for the body to break down. These are found in foods that are high in fibre and starches, such as brans, seeds, beans, lentils, peas, legumes, and some vegetables. It is considered that these are healthier due to the length of time it takes to break them down, and they are a better option than simple carbohydrates. These carbohydrates contain other vitamins and minerals and are therefore the healthier of the two options, but the truth is that it depends on your health history and whether you have any kind of insulin resistance or gut issue. If you do, carbohydrates of any kind, even complex carbs, are not your friend.

As insulin resistance is common in perimenopause, there can often be a period where women struggle to metabolize any carbohydrates at all and instead will feel as though they are piling on weight regardless of what they do. This would be when we recommend significantly reducing your intake of any carbohydrates. But this doesn't last forever: once your hormones have settled down post-menopause and your weight has stabilized, you can try reintroducing them carefully!

It would be remiss to discuss carbohydrates without talking about refined carbohydrates.

These are grain products that have been processed by a food manufacturer so that the whole grain is taken apart. The refining or milling process removes dietary fibre, vitamins, and minerals, meaning the carbs are not only processed "unnatural" foods but also often simple carbohydrates. They are often high in calories and when they are found in pre-packaged foods, they are commonly paired with seed oils.

Examples of refined carbs would be:

- pasta (especially white pasta)
- biscuits and pastries
- cakes and baked goods
- white bread
- baked desserts
- pizza dough.

Although many of us find these delicious, the combination of them being predominantly wheat, processed and refined, and paired with seed oils makes them a serious "triple threat" to our health and they must be eaten sparingly if we want to feel well!

Fibre

One of the subjects that muddies the water when discussing macronutrients is fibre, as people are confused about where it fits.

Predominantly fibre sits in the carbohydrate macronutrient category.

Fibre is also called roughage or bulk. Fibre is food the body can't digest or absorb. Unlike proteins, fats, or carbohydrates, fibre isn't broken down and digested.

There are two types of fibre: insoluble and soluble.

Insoluble fibre is found in vegetables, whole grains, and fruits. It adds bulk to the stool and appears to help food pass more quickly through the stomach and intestines.

Soluble fibre is found in oat bran, barley, nuts, seeds, beans, lentils, peas, and some fruits and vegetables. It attracts water and turns to a gel which slows down digestion. It helps hydrate the body and moves waste through your intestines. It slows down the absorption of sugars and reduces blood sugar spiking. It also binds with fatty acids and helps lower LDL cholesterol.

While fibre is important, we need to be mindful of the fact that although soluble fibre slows down blood sugar spiking, it is still a carbohydrate, and we can't be complacent about the destabilizing effects of carbohydrates on the Triangle of Hormonal Health.

Foods that combine macronutrients

This is a simplified way of looking at macronutrients as many foods contain a few of the macronutrients. For example, cheese and nuts contain protein and fat, and beans contain protein and carbohydrate.

Because of this, many vegetarians and vegans believe that they are eating protein when they eat beans, but they contain a much higher level of carbohydrates than protein. For example, 100g of chickpeas contain 19g of protein and 6g of fat, but they also contain a whopping 61g of carbohydrate. So, for the purposes of ensuring we are getting the right amount of protein and not too much carbohydrate, these sit very clearly in the carbohydrate category.

Additionally, protein can only be utilized fully once the food has been broken down. This is important to remember when we are looking at foods that are predominantly carbohydrates being used as a protein source because, as we said earlier, every time we put food in our mouth, we have a hormone response. In the case of foods like chickpeas, the initial hormone response will be for a carbohydrate. The body will only recognize the protein component much later. For all intents and purposes, therefore, when we eat chickpeas, the body acts as if it's getting carbohydrates, and the protein comes as a nice surprise later. In contrast, when we eat a pure protein source such as eggs, the body will instantly recognize it is eating protein and produce the hormones for protein. That is how we maintain good blood sugar balancing.

Macronutrient identification at a glance

Protein 115–250g*	Fat 2 tbsp*	Non-starchy carbohydrates unlimited	Starchy carbohydrates ½ cup*
All meat	Nuts	All cruciferous vegetables	All root vegetables
All fish	Cheese	Salad leaves	All fruits
Eggs	Seeds	Cucumbers	All grains
Tofu	Avocado	Non-root vegetables	All beans and legumes
Protein powders	Tallow and lard		Sweeteners such as honey, sugar, maple syrup
	Butter		Alcohol
	Cream		Sweet treats
	Olives and olive oil		Baked goods
	Coconut oil and milk		Pasta and bread

* Amount per meal.

Bioavailability of protein

There is another factor to consider here and that is how much protein we yield from the food we eat. This is called "bioavailability".

A quick look on Google shows us that proteins from animal foods such as meat, fish, and eggs score much higher on a "bioavailability index" (also called the Digested Indispensable Amino Acid Score, DIAAS) than proteins from plants such as rice protein, pea protein, or hemp protein.

What this means is that if you are eating a protein bar that says that it contains 16g of protein from plant proteins or nuts, you might only absorb

8g, whereas if that protein came from whey protein or another animal-based protein source, you might absorb around 12–14g.

This is why it is essential, at every meal, that we:

- prioritize protein
- don't fear fat
- cut carbs.

The PFC Food Strategy

There are thousands of different types of diets and food strategies, but where many fail is that they don't focus on the fact that every time we eat, we have a hormonal response, and the hormones can either spike or balance our blood sugars.

Balancing blood sugars is exactly what the PFC Food Strategy was created to do and is at the heart of all our food plans.

PFC was developed by renowned nutrition expert Mark Macdonald to overcome the issues in the food industry. The letters P, F, and C stand for the three "macronutrient" categories that every food falls into – protein, fat, and carbohydrate – and the idea is that every time we eat, we eat the right balance of all the macronutrients.

The PFC Food Strategy has similarities with the Paleo diet and the Zone diet. Like the Paleo diet, the PFC approach focuses on real, whole foods while removing inflammatory foods like bread, pasta, and grains that can interfere with optimal digestion, energy levels, and vitality. However, unlike the Paleo approach, the top priority is to focus on the individual and on eliminating the individual's food intolerances as part of the plan.

Perhaps the biggest difference between the PFC approach and the Paleo diet is the emphasis on timing. It is not just about eating the correct foods that our ancestors ate; when you eat those foods (or don't) plays a huge role in how your metabolism functions and how your brain and body work, too.

"PFC every three" is the term coined to refer to eating a combination of the three "macros" every 3–4 hours, from within an hour of waking up, until your head hits the pillow at night.

This keeps your blood sugar levels balanced, which is the key to everything from awesome energy levels, positive mood, improved mental clarity, and supported metabolism to vanished sugar cravings.

It is common to see people eating a Paleo diet without the right ratios of proteins, fats and carbohydrates, leading to blood sugar imbalances.

PFC is a great baseline diet plan as many people are not having protein at each meal. For example, a diet of porridge for breakfast, a cheese sandwich for lunch, and spaghetti bolognese for dinner has no protein at breakfast or lunch, and is high in starchy carbohydrates, so it isn't a balanced representation of each macronutrient.

For a PFC Food Strategy sheet and recipes, visit www.hormone-wellness. co.uk.

PFC rules

The PFC Food Strategy

Protein 115–250g*	Fat 2 tbsp*	Non-starchy carbohydrates unlimited	Starchy carbohydrates ½ cup*
All meat	Avocado	All non-starchy vegetables and salad leaves	All root vegetables
All fish	Coconut oil, cream, and milk		Grains and beans
Eggs			Legumes
Tofu	Olives and olive oil		All fruit
Protein powders	Organic mayonnaise		honey and maple syrup
	Dripping, suet, and lard		Dark chocolate
	Butter		Small alcoholic drink (125 ml)
	Cheese		
	Nuts and seeds		
	Gluten-free pork scratchings		
	Tahini		

Amount per meal.

- Choose a protein and fat source for each meal.

- Protein needs to be 125–250g per meal (fist-size portion).

- Add as many non-starchy carbs (salad and greens) as you like but only have *one* starchy carbohydrate in a half-cup portion per meal (e.g. a small potato). Non-starchy carbohydrates will not spike blood sugars, whereas starchy carbohydrates do, which is why they are limited.

- Fat intake is important. Eat 1–2 tablespoons per meal depending on the size of your protein portion. It depends on appetite so for the smaller protein portion it would be 1 tablespoon of fat for the larger portion it would be 2 tablespoons of fat.

- If you have sleep difficulties, have a bedtime snack of a few mouthfuls of a fat and carb combination, 20 minutes before sleep. This can help improve sleep if sleep disturbances are due to unstable blood sugars.

- Drink plenty of water – a minimum of 2 litres per day (can include herbal tea).

- Eat regularly every three hours. Eat three meals and three snacks per day.

- Exercise. Even going for a walk improves blood sugar stability.

- Avoid stimulants and irritants such as caffeine, alcohol, and nicotine.

- If carbohydrates are indulged in (e.g. a piece of chocolate or a glass of wine), offset the sugar with fat (e.g. add coconut cream, olives, or nuts).

CASE STUDY: "T", 46
Symptoms

- Struggling to lose weight

- Intense three-day headache pain ahead of bleed

- Autoimmune skin condition

- Regularly experiencing anaemia

- Fatigue and rarely feeling energized

- Struggling with excessive hunger

- IBS symptoms after eating

- Too tired to work out

- Poor sleep

Current diet

- **Breakfast:** Yoghurt and fruit or eggs and toast or a croissant

- **Lunch:** Pizza or sandwich

- **Dinner:** Meat and vegetables, homemade curry, or stew. One night a week, a takeaway such as burger or Chinese takeaway

- **Snacks:** fruit, crisps, toast, crumpet

Current supplements

- Magnesium

- Menopause support

What was recommended and why?

- Remove wheat from the diet. It was being consumed up to four times a day, which is contributing to symptoms and inflammation. Wheat is also an antinutrient, stopping the absorption of iron.

- Eat PFC at every meal as diet looks as though it is lacking in consistent protein and is carb-heavy.

Results after 12 weeks

- Reduced autoimmune flare-ups

- No IBS issues

- Lost 7kg

- Increased energy and improved sleep

The PFC diet is very different to the diet that is promoted by the NHS and the standard Western medical approach.

The medically approved diet

In the UK, the medically approved diet is called the Eatwell Guide, which is ironic because it is anything but eating well.

The Eatwell Guide says that most of our meals should be based on starchy carbohydrates such as pasta, which is astonishingly bad advice given the obesity epidemic that is happening because we are consuming too many carbohydrates.

Eatwell considers legumes such as lentils to be a protein source, when we've clearly demonstrated above that they are predominantly a carbohydrate. Eatwell also insists that margarine is a good fat when we have so much evidence to the contrary with regard to vegetable oils.

The Eatwell plate is highly outdated, and many charities and organizations such as the Public Health Collaboration are lobbying for it to be changed. There have been inroads made with the Freshwell app, which challenges these outdated views and which many doctors are now referring patients to instead of the traditional NHS information.

The importance of reading food labels

Learning to identify what is in the food you are buying is an important step in making conscious food choices. We can do that by learning to read food labels. Many foods claim to be healthy or high in protein, but when we learn to look at the label, we see that they are, in fact, higher in carbs than protein (many protein bars are guilty of this). It isn't always obvious whether a food is counted as a protein, fat, or carbohydrate – for example, yogurt can fall into any of the categories, and the only way to establish which one it fits is by checking the nutritional data.

We do this by looking at the back of the packet for the table showing nutritional amounts per serving, per 100ml, or per 100g.

Ignoring everything else, just look for how much protein, fat, or carbohydrate is in that item per serving, 100ml, or 100g.

For the purposes of the PFC food plan, we aren't interested in how many of the carbohydrates are "sugars", just the overall amount of carbohydrate.

Let's take, for example, baked beans. These are commonly thought of as a protein, but when we look at the nutritional data, we can see that this is far from the truth.

	Per 100g	Per ½ can	%RI*
Energy	339kJ	703kJ	–
	81kcal	168kcal	8%
Fat	0.4g	0.7g	1%
– of which saturates	<0.1g	0.1g	<1%
Carbohydrates	15.5g	32.1g	12%
– of which sugars	4.3g	8.9g	10%
Fibre	3.9g	8.0g	–
Protein	4.8g	10.0g	20%
Salt	0.6g	1.3g	21%

*RI per serving. Reference intake of an average adult (8400kJ/2000kcal

Servings per can – 2

DIAGRAM 26 – THE NUTRITIONAL DATA OF BAKED BEANS

When we ignore all the other information and focus solely on the macronutrients, we can see that per 100g, there is 0.4g of fat, 15.5g of carbohydrate, and 4.8g of protein. The carbohydrate content here is vast in comparison to the other macronutrients, so this is counted as a carbohydrate.

Do not worry about counting calories at this stage. It is more important to be eating real food in a balanced way and avoiding food intolerances.

Another aspect of reading food labels is to be mindful of noticing when you don't recognize an ingredient. If you look at the label and it resembles a chemistry lesson with long names that you don't understand, put it back. This is an indication that this food is ultra-processed, full of synthetic chemicals, and not fit for human health.

It is shocking when you realize that the "free from" aisle is positioned as being healthy but often contains foods that are filled with chemicals and have been processed so much that the body doesn't recognize them as food. This is the same in many health food shops – they are full of ultra-processed, packaged foods that are marketed in a way that makes us believe they are a better option.

The importance of organic

The term "organic" refers to the process of how certain foods are produced. Organic foods have been grown or farmed without the use of toxic chemicals, hormones, or antibiotics.

To be labelled organic, a food product must be free of artificial food additives. This includes artificial sweeteners, preservatives, colouring, flavouring, and monosodium glutamate (MSG).

Organic farming tends to improve soil quality and the conservation of groundwater. It also reduces pollution and may be better for the environment.

Studies have found that organic foods generally contain higher levels of antioxidants and certain micronutrients, such as vitamin C, zinc, and iron. Organically grown crops have also been shown to have lower levels of nitrate.

Organic milk and dairy products contain higher levels of omega-3 fatty acids and slightly higher amounts of iron, vitamin E, and some carotenoids. A review of 67 studies found that organic meat contained higher levels of omega-3 fatty acids and slightly lower levels of saturated fats than conventional meat.[1] One study found that levels of the heavy metal cadmium were 48 per cent lower in organic produce.[2]

The Dirty Dozen and Clean Fifteen

Buying organic is optimal. However, for some it can be price prohibitive or unavailable. Knowing which foods to prioritize when purchasing organic is helpful. The Environmental Working Group in the USA has identified the Dirty Dozen[3] – the worse contaminated fruits and vegetables – and the Clean Fifteen[4] – the least contaminated. Although these lists represent food sold in the USA, it's likely to be a similar story in the UK and Europe. These do change every year but for illustrative purposes in 2024 the lists were as follows.

The Dirty Dozen

1. Strawberries
2. Spinach
3. Kale, collard, and mustard greens
4. Grapes
5. Peaches
6. Pears
7. Nectarines
8. Apples
9. Bell and hot peppers
10. Cherries
11. Blueberries
12. Green beans

The Clean Fifteen

1. Avocados
2. Sweetcorn
3. Pineapples
4. Onions
5. Papaya
6. Peas (frozen)
7. Asparagus
8. Honeydew melon
9. Kiwifruit
10. Cabbage
11. Mushrooms
12. Mangoes
13. Sweet potatoes
14. Watermelon
15. Carrots

There are other ways to make eating organic cheaper.

Try growing your own fruit, vegetables, and herbs. You can grow herbs and sprouts on your windowsill if you don't have a garden.

If you buy organic meat, use every part of it. The skin and bones can be used to make a nutritious stock along with the vegetable peelings and leaves that you would otherwise discard.

Supermarkets sometimes have offers on organic fruit and vegetables, so be flexible and buy what's on offer at a good price. Frozen organic foods may be less expensive.

Myth busting

The health industry is full of myths, and we are passionate about exploring the research behind the claims to see what is real and what is false.

The following is a small list of health myth traps we have fallen into ourselves in the past and that we commonly hear clients talking about.

Juicing

The juicing diet trend has increased in popularity over the years, but its effectiveness is questionable. Juicing is the process of extracting the liquid from fruits and vegetables, while removing the fibre. This can be done by hand or with a motor-driven juicer.

In the past, mixed fruit and vegetable juices were all the rage, but more recently there is a big trend for having celery juice daily.

There are some pros to juicing (it's not all bad). Fruit and vegetables are rich in vitamins and minerals – for example, celery juice contains vitamin A, vitamin C, vitamin K, folate, calcium, potassium, sodium, magnesium, phosphorus, electrolytes, and water.

However, when fruit and veg are juiced, they lose their fibre, without which we have a quicker blood sugar response. Devoid of this fibre, fruit or vegetable juice is just sugar water with added vitamins and materials. Fibre helps you to feel fuller, supports healthy cholesterol levels, and feeds the good bacteria in your gut, so it doesn't make much sense to remove it.

On top of this, specifically in the case of celery juice, celery is one of the most common allergens on the planet. It's so common that it legally must be listed in bold as an ingredient on food packets. How telling people to drink it daily as a broad-brush cure-all is beyond us. In fact, we commonly see people having adrenal symptoms after drinking it, in line with food intolerance reactions. Added to these issues, if juices aren't consumed rapidly or have been pasteurised (in the case of shop bought juices), many of the beneficial nutrients are destroyed.

Some use juicing as a detox, but there are no scientific studies showing that replacing solid food with juice will detoxify the body. As we explored when we discussed the liver, our body is able to get rid of toxins on its own, and when we remove protein from our diet, we inhibit this in-built system.

Many vegetables are high in oxalates. Oxalates are organic compounds found in leafy greens, vegetables, fruits, cocoa, nuts, and seeds, and they contribute to inflammation.

Several studies have shown patients developing oxalate-induced acute kidney failure due to the consumption of oxalate-rich fruit and vegetable juices.[5]

Vegan diets

In general, the vegan diet is promoted as being very healthy and best for the planet. However, there is a lot of "greenwashing" happening around this dietary philosophy that doesn't stack up under closer examination. A great book (and film) that explores this in more depth than we can cover here is *Sacred Cow* by Diana Rogers and Robb Wolf.[6]

Vegans choose not to consume dairy, eggs, meat, fish, or any other products of animal origin. Some vegans are very mindful of their food and supplement accordingly. However, we have worked with a great many unwell vegans, and this is because the biggest problem with a vegan diet is the lack of nutrition.

Nutrients that are not present in plant foods:

- preformed vitamin A
- creatine
- vitamin B12
- carnosine
- taurine
- iron
- EPA and DHA omega-3 fatty acids
- vitamin D3
- vitamin K2 (MK-4 subtype).

Nutrients that are low in plant foods:

- protein
- heme iron
- zinc
- iodine
- methionine
- leucine
- choline
- glycine
- co-enzyme Q10
- active vitamin B6 (pyridoxal-5-phosphate)
- vitamin B2 (riboflavin).

These nutrients are required for hormone health, blood sugar balancing, digestive function, and immune responses.

Our experience is that most vegans (and vegetarians) must prioritize eating protein at every meal. As we've shown previously, the bioavailability of plant proteins is significantly lower than animal-based proteins, so focusing on getting these in wherever possible is essential.

The other issue with a diet full of plant food is that plants have a significant number of defence chemicals to stop predators from eating them. These defence chemicals can cause some serious inflammation and intolerance reactions. Having a diet saturated in them isn't the best idea for health.

A common quote we hear is that when people turn vegetarian, they swap meat for cheese, and when they turn vegan, they swap cheese for bread. With the global issues we are seeing surrounding wheat intolerance, this does not equal optimal health.

Ultimately, with all food fads it comes back to avoiding the hype and emotional pull towards the claims and coming back to some basic questions to help us work out if a food is beneficial, such as:

- Did our ancestors need this to thrive?

- Does it require processing or specialist equipment?

- Does it come from a lab?

- Does it need an advert or a stack of propaganda to convince me to buy it?

The best way for us to eat is to get back to our ancestral roots and eat a species-appropriate diet.

TAKE-HOME MESSAGE

The first step to eating in a way that balances your hormones and supports full body health is to eat protein, fat, and carbohydrates in the right amount at every meal.

Give up wheat and sugar. Avoid ultra-processed food. Learn to read labels and make yourself aware of what you are eating.

This approach has changed the lives and health of thousands of people. However, if after a month of doing it, you haven't achieved your health goals, then it's time to move on to the next stage...

— CHAPTER 14 —

Navigating symptoms with a staged approach

We have seen miracles happen when women take control of their diet, remove food intolerances, and eat more protein. However, as we have discussed in depth, many women experiencing a challenging menopause have navigated other symptoms throughout their lives. In these situations, we commonly need a more dynamic approach.

This is because their symptoms, such as immune reactions, fatigue, and IBS, are often the tip of the iceberg with relation to hormone imbalances.

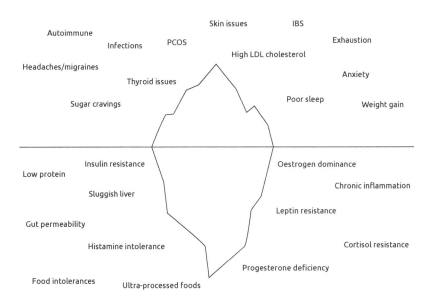

DIAGRAM 27 – THE SYMPTOMS ICEBERG, SHOWING THE SYMPTOMS THAT PRESENT WITH THE UNDERLYING CAUSES

Utilizing the processes we've outlined previously will begin the journey of getting below the surface and promoting gut health, liver support, and hormone balancing. However, if you have spent years of your life yo-yo dieting, eating processed food, and being stressed to the max, this is going to take some time to repair. In some cases, to reduce the symptoms that are obvious at the tip of the iceberg we need to explore what is happening below the surface and to work on the causes.

These "further steps" are purposefully designed food strategies that work at the root of specific issues.

The food strategy pathway

As soon as you dive into research in the conflicting and confusing world of nutrition, you start to learn about various food strategies, targeting different issues. Some of these have been medically adopted, such as low-FODMAP for IBS and gut issues. Another example of a popular food strategy would be the autoimmune Paleo (AIP), which is aimed at reducing inflammation for people with autoimmune conditions.

Although these strategies are now quite commonplace, the research behind some of the foods and approaches now conflicts with new research that has come to light, and the reported results are often mixed. But what is clear from the research, our clinical observations, and our own journeys is that our food choices very definitely play a role in how we can manage and navigate symptoms.

Our food strategy pathway is based on much of the research behind these existing food plans, combined with other cutting-edge research and information, and the removal of foods that have other health issues associated with them. For example, low-FODMAP encourages the use of margarine and sweeteners, which, as we have discussed previously, can wreak havoc with our blood sugars, and the AIP allows a lot of fruit, which can be a problem for people with gut issues. Neither food strategy insists that protein is eaten in each meal, which means you could adhere strictly to both plans but still not experience symptom relief because the underlying hormonal imbalances aren't being corrected.

Our food intolerance hierarchy is rooted in AIP and FODMAP but without the need to comply with these strict full-diet plans. We believe that the "sweet spot" is being able to eliminate as few foods as possible to ensure minimal disruption to an enjoyable lifestyle. Why remove all gluten if all symptoms are resolved just by giving up wheat? If barley, rye, and spelt can be consumed without any adverse effect, then why do we need to remove them?

For some people, however, the reality is that their bodies are in an inflammatory response and need more extreme strategies. We know all too well how tough and unfair that can feel. We are those people!

In our experience, someone's desire to resolve the issue is directly proportionate to how badly the issue affects them. In other words, if it isn't affecting us that badly, we are probably unlikely to want to commit to an extreme way of eating to resolve it (unless we are truly dedicated health fanatics who love experimenting with nutrition). One of our favourite questions is "How bad does it have to get before you change it?"

The food strategy pathway has been created to give you the understanding of when and how to move forward if you aren't getting the results you want.

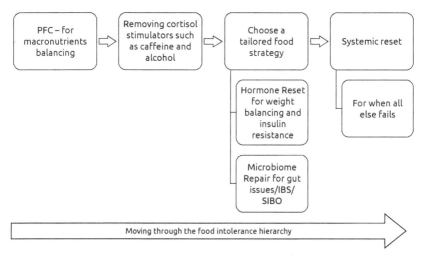

DIAGRAM 28 – THE FOOD STRATEGY PATHWAY

We always start at the beginning with PFC and removing food intolerances in the order of the food intolerance hierarchy for a period of 6–8 weeks. If, however, you aren't getting symptom relief, we now move to the next most appropriate food strategy: we need to drill more into either hormone balancing or gut repair. If, after a few months of working with these food plans, you still haven't improved, it's time to pull out all the stops and get stuck into the full elimination plan: the Systemic Reset.

Let's look at each strategy individually.

Hormone Reset Food Strategy

Benefits: Improving insulin sensitivity and weight loss.

Focuses on: Intermittent fasting, low carb, fat reduction.

Prerequisites: PFC for a minimum of a month to ensure baseline blood sugar balancing followed by two weeks of PFC minus starchy carbs

Many, many women struggle with weight gain and insulin resistance during menopause. If eating PFC for 4–6 weeks isn't enough to start weight loss and blood sugar stabilizing, we would recommend removing any starchy carbohydrates from the diet for two weeks and monitoring any change and improvement. Starchy carbohydrates can be metabolized as quickly as and sometimes more quickly than sugar, which means that they can rapidly increase blood sugar levels after eating and contribute to insulin resistance.

If removing starchy carbohydrates isn't enough to kick-start weight loss, we recommend the hormone food strategy. There are three focuses in this strategy:

- removing starchy carbohydrates
- reducing fat
- intermittent fasting.

This is a short-term focused approach to balance the hormone rollercoaster that contributes to weight gain in perimenopause. It must only be done for three weeks, and then the client must return to PFC for one week before going back to another three-week round of the Hormone Reset Food Strategy. This helps avoid the body going into a starvation mode and storing weight.

Short-term is the emphasis here because low-carbohydrate intake can depress the thyroid, which can lead to further weight issues, and low-fat stops our hormone production, which is why it is only recommended to adopt this strategy for three weeks at a time.

Although we are still eating fat, we are eating much less of it. Approximately one teaspoon per meal instead of two tablespoons. Fat is essential, and we don't want to undo all the hard work we have put in to making you realize how much we need it; however, the truth is that for some women, the liver struggles during menopause and can't metabolize it well, so the middle ground is to make sure we are eating a whole-food fat source but being sparing with the quantity.

Avoid: Food intolerances and starchy carbohydrates: fruit, root vegetables, grains, beans, legumes, sweeteners (except stevia), alcohol, sweet treats.

Ensure: Protein, fats, and carbs are eaten at every meal!

We are also encouraging women to eat only twice a day with this strategy and to follow an eight-hour eating window – for example, eating a brunch at 11 a.m. and a dinner at 7 p.m. but avoiding snacking in between. This two-meals-a-day, intermittent fast has had a huge amount of positive research. With all fasting, we recommend speaking to your GP or healthcare provider if you have any underlying conditions that prevent this approach.

The combination of the fasting with low carb and low fat is great for losing weight while rebalancing underlying hormonal imbalances.

We also recommend avoiding soy because it is highly oestrogenic, so tofu should be eliminated.

Timeframe: Three weeks on, one week off until the goal weight has been reached; returning to PFC is the maintenance recommendation.

The Hormone Reset Food Strategy

Protein 115g only*	Fat 1 tsp only*	Non-starchy carbohydrates 2 cups only*	Starchy carbohydrates
All meat All fish Eggs Protein powders (non-soy or whey)	Nuts Cheese Seeds Avocado Dripping and lard Butter Cream Olives and olive oil Coconut oil and milk	All cruciferous vegetables Salad leaves and vegetables Non-root vegetables	None

Amount per meal.

CASE STUDY: "C", 40

Symptoms: C had been eating a PFC diet for months but, due to perimenopause, could not get her weight to shift.

History: She had put on a total of three stone in two years.

Results: After committing to the Hormone Reset Food Strategy, C lost all the weight in a timeframe of eight months. She then returned to PFC eating and would do a round of the Hormone Reset Food Strategy if she felt her weight fluctuate. She had maintained the weight loss after seven years.

Microbiome Repair Food Strategy

Benefits: Reducing intestinal permeability, reducing gut inflammation by eliminating exposure to allergens and intolerances.

Focuses on: FODMAP exclusion including fruit, and elimination of all food intolerances in the hierarchy, including dairy. No raw food.

Prerequisites: PFC for one month with removal of all food intolerances in the hierarchy.

The Microbiome Repair Food Strategy takes the PFC principles further by layering a gut microbiome support strategy on top of it.

The strategy incorporates three areas:

- the science behind PFC for blood sugar balancing

- selected FODMAP exclusion including allium (garlic, onions, and leeks)

- food intolerance elimination of grains, nuts, and nightshades (similar to the Autoimmune Protocol).

FODMAP stands for fermentable oligosaccharides, disaccharides, monosaccharides, and polyols, which basically means the sugars that upset the small intestine and are not easily absorbed. The FODMAP diet was first made popular in the early 2000s by Dr Peter Gibson and Dr Sue Shepherd. It is a diet that is prescribed by medical dieticians and limits foods that have been shown to aggravate the gut and cause IBS symptoms. Some people have great results by simply cutting out FODMAPs, but there are many compliance issues with the diet, and it doesn't consider other factors contributing to digestive issues such as blood sugar and stress imbalances or food intolerances.

We have created a plan combining low-FODMAP with the Autoimmune Protocol because this plan was ground-breaking in its focus on eliminating intolerances and whole-food eating, overlaid with the principles of PFC (i.e. making sure to eat protein and fat with every meal to keep the hormonal responses balanced).

A key part of this plan is not eating raw food. Raw food can be very hard for the stomach and intestines to process, so it is recommended that all vegetables and fruits are steamed or cooked. It is therefore not advised to eat salads unless they are made with cooked or lightly steamed vegetables.

We also recommend avoiding fruit. SIBO is a common cause of IBS, and we want to avoid the sugar aspect of fruit feeding SIBO while doing this repair food strategy.

We recommend doing this strategy for three months and then assessing progress. If symptoms have abated, return carefully to PFC, reintroducing foods one at a time to see if they are contributing to digestive issues.

The Microbiome Repair Food Strategy

Protein 115–250g*	Fat 2 tbsp*	Non-starchy carbohydrates unlimited	Starchy carbohydrates ½ cup*
All meat	Avocado	All non-starchy vegetables	All root vegetables
All fish	Coconut oil and milk		Maple syrup
Eggs			Honey
Tofu	Olives and olive oil		
Protein powders	Tallow and lard		
	Butter		

* Amount per meal.

Avoid: Raw food, fruit, nightshades, all grains, beans, and legumes.

Ensure: Protein, fats, and carbs are eaten at every meal!

Timeframe: Three months, then assess symptom progress and return to PFC minus intolerances or progress to Systemic Reset Food Strategy.

CASE STUDY: "N", 36

Symptoms: Regular heavy periods with hunger and acne breakouts, sugar cravings, bowel pain with bloating, demotivated and lethargic with chronic anxiety.

History: Prior to eating PFC, N ate a carb-heavy diet of pasta, bread, refined carbohydrates, and fruit. After eating PFC for 12 weeks, her symptoms improved but didn't clear entirely. It was recommended she try the Microbiome Repair Food Strategy.

Results: Within four weeks, her anxiety, acne, sleep, and energy were vastly improved. She returned to PFC eating.

Systemic Reset Food Strategy

Benefits: Anti-inflammatory, gut repair, immune resetting.

Focuses on: Full elimination and re-introduction.

Prerequisites: PFC and food intolerance elimination but it's not worked sufficiently.

This strategy is an option for those who are not experiencing benefit from the previous food strategies and have a more complicated health picture, with numerous unresolved underlying health issues.

The Systemic Reset Food Strategy is based on the carnivore diet. The principle is that by eating good-quality meat, meat fats such as dripping and suet, plus organ meats, fish, and eggs (if tolerated), while reducing all potentially inflammatory foods, we are able to heal the gut and relieve the immune system. These inflammatory foods include all plant foods, dairy, vegetable oils, and ultra-processed foods.

This approach has been pioneered by the likes of Dr Shawn Baker, Dr Paul Saladino, Dr Anthony Chafee, and Dr Kevin Stocks.

While this may sound counterintuitive to the messages we have been blasted with since childhood such as "eat your greens" and "an apple a day keeps the doctor at bay", the research is truly mind-blowing, and the reports of the millions of people who have chosen to eat this way and alleviated major health issues are astonishing.

Many, many pioneering doctors are utilizing the principles of the carnivore diet to offer cutting-edge treatments for a variety of deeply complex conditions. Dr Georgia Ede, author and Metabolic Psychiatrist at Harvard University Health Services discusses in depth how removing plant foods benefits historically medicated mental health conditions,[1] while Dr Zsófia Clemens has had the most astonishing results working with people with autoimmune disease and specific cancers with a strict carnivore diet.[2] As a little aside, we have both tried every food strategy and diet possible, and although many things helped a bit, nothing worked as effectively as the carnivore diet. We have truly walked the path and know the challenges but have also reaped the benefits.

This diet highlights the fact that there are toxic chemicals inherent in plants to prevent them from being eaten by predators. Surprisingly, most of the plants that are supposed to be "good for you" have the same toxins as plants that will kill you. It's simply the dose of the toxin that is different. Rhubarb leaves, for instance, are commonly known as being deadly because they contain a high amount of a pesticide called oxalic acid. But kale and spinach have the exact same toxin, only in smaller amounts. In fact, almost all plants have oxalic acid in varying amounts as a defence mechanism to keep insects and other pests from eating them. Oxalates are dangerous to humans as well as pests, and exposure to them in everyday foods, such as spinach and tea, have caused previously healthy people to go into kidney failure from an overdose of these toxic compounds.

It has only been our human ingenuity in figuring out how to process plants that has allowed us to mitigate their toxins sufficiently to eat them. For example:

- Wheat is indigestible uncooked or unsprouted.

- The lectins in beans and legumes can be deadly if left uncooked.

- Cassava (tapioca) contains deadly levels of cyanide unless specially prepared.

- Potatoes contain the toxin solanine, which needs to be cooked to become inactive.

- Acorns and olives need to be extensively soaked to remove tannins.

- Cashews contain urushiol, which will cause severe chemical burns unless deactivated by cooking.

And as we've touched on previously, many plants contain "antinutrients" that stop vitamins and minerals from being absorbed:

- Phytates in grains and beans block zinc absorption.

- Lectins in legumes and grains block mineral absorption.

- Oxalates in green leafy vegetables and nuts block calcium and iron.

- Goitrogens present in brassicas like broccoli block thyroid hormones.

- Tannins found in tea, chocolate, and wine block iron absorption.

- Polyphenols found in brightly coloured plants block iron absorption.

Once we start diving down the rabbit hole into this research, we quickly come across language such as "species-appropriate diet". This is an explanation about how we evolved to eat. As omnivores, humans *can* eat anything, but this diet focuses on what we *ought* to be eating for real health and vitality based on our ancestral roots.

Although we might love a nice roast chicken on a Sunday, if you think about when we would be out hunting as a tribe, we would have needed a lot of chickens to feed, say, a dozen people, whereas you would only need one goat or sheep. It would make energetic sense to focus the attention of multiple hunters on the one bigger kill to ensure there was enough food to feed everyone. Our diet was therefore heavy in ruminant meat, also called red meat. Meats like chicken or pork are also renowned for carrying disease and therefore need careful cooking, which may not have been possible, but ruminant meat can be eaten raw if it is fresh.

Fruit and vegetables were only available if in season and would only be available if they were stumbled across during a hunt, so our exposure to them would have been minimal, and there was certainly not enough available to feed a tribe. The kill was revered, and nothing was wasted. Today, we call this "eating nose to tail".

A nose-to-tail meat approach includes high-quality red meat, but it also includes organ meats, connective tissue (a good source of collagen), and some consideration of the fat-to-protein ratio. This strategy is best adopted to include nutrient-dense foods such as fatty cuts of meat, grass-fed minced beef, eggs, seafood, and sources of animal fat like butter, lard, dripping, or suet.

Mainstream thinking would suggest that eating a lot of red meat would lead to cardiovascular disease, but this just isn't true when we look at the evidence shown by our ancestral health, the health of indigenous hunter-gatherer tribes still in existence, and the positive changes in health markers of people who have committed to this diet (Claire's cholesterol dropped from 6.4 to 5.8 within a year of committing to carnivore).

What appears more likely is that insulin resistance is the main driver of plaque formation in our arteries because our blood becomes more "sticky" when we can't remove the sugar from our bloodstream, rather than LDL itself, and this diet actively avoids foods that create an insulin response.

This diet isn't without its challenges, however.

Many people (ourselves included) need time to process that many of our commonly held beliefs around vegetables are incorrect and that broccoli and kale are not our friends.

It can feel restrictive and takes some forward planning. Knowing the tips for what to eat in an emergency and how to eat when travelling can take time to figure out.

There is a transition period for the gut microbiome to detox, which can take a few weeks and during which we can feel unwell (commonly called "carnivore flu").

It can be done incorrectly, and people can feel quite unwell.

It can be expensive if you've not planned well, but it is comparable to other ways of eating when you do plan and buy in large amounts from independent butchers.

Exponents of the diet say that once you have got into a groove, it is easy and doesn't feel restrictive, and for many people, eating a steak for breakfast feels like a treat every day.

However, this dietary approach is still relatively new, and the research is unfolding. One of our favourite evangelists, Dr Paul Saladino, reversed his position on being 100 per cent carnivore and now promotes what he calls an "animal-based" approach, and his research into why is compelling.

Ultimately, for truly great health, we do benefit from having carbohydrates in our diet, and people who have had a history of long-term hormone dysregulation and gut issues very much benefit from having some carbohydrates in the diet.

Dr Saladino spent time with the Hadza people, a protected hunter-gatherer indigenous ethnic group of Tanzania. He discovered that while their diet is predominantly meat, offal, and eggs, it also includes seasonal fruit and honey, plus raw dairy.

The research on fruit shows us that the fruit is the part of the plant that is safer to eat. It wants us eating this part so we can distribute the seeds, which is evolutionarily beneficial to the plant's survival.

Our Systemic Reset Food Strategy therefore utilizes the best of both approaches and offers a two-phased approach.

Many people are concerned about making sure they have enough vitamins and fibre on this plan. Our fat-soluble vitamins come from the meat fats, our water-soluble vitamins are included in part in the meat itself but mostly in the offal, and our fibre comes from eating all the meat, including the chewy bits. Nose-to-tail eating offers a full spectrum of nutrition.

- **Phase 1: Full carnivore** – to remove all allergens and intolerances and offer a total gut and immune system reset.

- **Phase 2: Animal-based** – low-toxin plant foods (fruits and root), A2 casein, and raw dairy, with raw honey reintroduced.

Phase 1: Full carnivore

The Systemic Reset Food Strategy – Phase 1: Full carnivore

Protein	Fat	Non-starchy carbohydrates	Starchy carbohydrates
All meat	Ghee	None	None
All fish	Suet		
Eggs (if tolerated)	Lard		
Offal	Dripping		
Bone broth			

Avoid: All plant-based food and all sugars, alcohol, all vegetable oils, and ultra-processed food. Don't do this without spending time researching it at the very least. We recommend working with a coach trained in this food strategy.

Ensure: You eat enough! The calculations for this swap between imperial and metric and can be quite confusing, but the easiest way is to divide your weight by 100 to find out how much meat to eat in a day. Ie someone weighing 75kg would eat .75kg of meat per day.

Then add a decimal point after the 1 to find how much meat to eat a day. In the example, 120lbs body weight = 1.20lbs of uncooked meat. And then you can use an online converter if your meat is sold in kilos. In this case, 1.2lbs of fresh meat is 0.544kg of meat per day.

Someone weighing 75kg would be 165lbs which equals 1.65lbs of fresh meat needed per day or 0.75kg.

Also ensure you are prepared and have snacks. Finding sources of foods that work on this plan is helpful. Foods like sugar-free biltong and wheat-free pork scratchings are great. Fast-food restaurants can do burger patties without the bun and sauces as an emergency option when eating on the run.

Offal is an important component of this plan. If you can't bear eating offal, we recommend buying desiccated offal supplements.

Timeframe: Three months ideally before moving to animal-based.

Phase 2: Animal-based PFC – reintroducing non-meat fats, fruit, roots, and raw honey

The Systemic Reset Food Strategy – Phase 2: Animal-based PFC

Protein 115–250g*	Fat 2tbsp*	Non-starchy carbohydrates ½–1 cup*	Starchy carbohydrates ½–1 cup*
All meat	Ghee	Artichokes	All root vegetables
All fish	Suet	Cucumber	All *seasonal* fruit
Eggs (if tolerated)	Lard	Courgette and marrow	Raw honey
Offal	Dripping	Lettuce	White rice
Bone broth	Suet	Sauerkraut and pickles	(occasional)
	Avocado	(if no bloating occurs)	
	Coconut oil		
	Olives and olive oil		
	A2 casein and raw dairy		

* Amount per meal.

Avoid: Reintroducing everything at once. Try one thing at a time and slowly build up. Alcohol is also to be avoided (for the most part). If alcohol or other foods are consumed (e.g. on holiday), consider a week of full carnivore if symptoms return.

Ensure: Honey *must* be raw and unfiltered. Raw honey does not spike blood sugars, but standard supermarket honey (including Manuka honey) is boiled and pasteurized, and this becomes a high-fructose syrup, which causes blood sugar spiking.

Timeframe: Unlimited.

Troubleshooting with the Systemic Reset Food Strategy

There are often some adjustment issues for the first 2–3 weeks, but if you are experiencing issues for longer than this, you may be eating a food that doesn't suit you.

If you adopt this way of eating and are not getting results, question whether you have meat food intolerances such as beef or chicken. Some people do not digest these foods well.

Question the origin of the meat source. There is a big difference in omega 6 content in farmed grain-fed animals and grass-fed animals. Find suppliers that are careful about feeding animals a species-appropriate diet!

Ensure you are eating enough fat in the forms of bone broth and fatty cuts of meat.

Slow-cooked meat and soups for digestive disorders are useful. These are easy to digest as they are well broken down and not chewy like a steak or a roasted joint of meat.

Bone broth can be very healing for intestinal permeability. If you have a reaction to broth, it may be a histamine response due to SIBO. This can also happen with aged meats. In this case, avoid bone broth and ensure you eat non-aged meats.

We don't recommend launching yourself into this strategy straight from a typical Western diet. Start with PFC and work through the food intolerance hierarchy.

If you have a history of eating disorders, please work with a coach or practitioner.

Half a teaspoon of apple cider vinegar in water before or during a meal can dramatically improve digestion. Digestive aid supplements can also help.

Watch out for going too low-carb if you have a thyroid condition. A clue that your carbs are too low is not being able to sleep.

Starting with a 'standard portion' is a great place to start to gauge whether or not hunger is the same or increasing/decreasing on the high protein approach.

CASE STUDY: "J", 44
Symptoms

- **Fatigue:** Mild to moderate ME/chronic fatigue symptoms, progressed slowly over 5–6 years. Struggling to walk for longer than 10–15 mins without a break and almost housebound. Can only work part-time, remotely. Used to be able to tolerate light yoga, long walks, and light jogs.

- **Unintentional weight loss:** Weight at first appointment was 45kg, down from 62kg two years prior. Medical tests do not show anything clinically wrong.

- **Digestive issues:** Gradually worsened. No longer able to eat enough calories. Overeating causes digestive pain "flare-ups" for days, and no dietary interventions have managed to solve this. J was not able to digest eating more than a certain "threshold" – a feeling of the intestines shutting down. Symptoms included distension, pulsing, bloating, and maybe diarrhoea too, along with feeling weak. J would then need to skip 1–3 subsequent meals over the next few days before things normalized.

- **Chronic migraine:** Struggled for years but very successfully managed by monthly injections.

Health history

J had worked with nutritionists and practitioners and had been through a variety of gastrointestinal testing via the NHS and multiple functional tests with no cause found. J subsequently had tried a variety of food strategies including several years on a whole-food PFC-style diet – no refined sugars or grains, but use of non-caloric sweeteners. Tried omitting eggs and dairy to no effect. Weight was decreasing and fatigue increasing. Always ate three meals a day, although portions became smaller over the years as symptoms, weight loss and fatigue increased.

J then progressed to the Autoimmune Protocol diet and adhered to the recommendations, but was still undereating and even felt there was a worsening of digestive and fatigue symptoms.

J was informed by their previous practitioner that there was nothing else that could be offered to them. J then did some research and discovered the carnivore diet, but tried this without support and was struggling to navigate it so reached out for coaching.

J was on a broad spectrum of supplements that are "traditional" in their approach and would have been what we would have recommended historically:

- adult multivitamins and minerals

- digestive enzymes with every meal

- betaine HCL with big meals

- adrenal glandular

- vitamin D (5000 iu)

- vitamin C (ascorbic acid – 1g/day).

What was recommended
J was a perfect candidate for the carnivore-inspired Systemic Reset Food Strategy. J is disciplined with compliance and committed to working through a process. They had also tried everything else to no avail.

Results after 16 weeks
J gained 10kg, felt a dramatic change in energy and digestive resilience, and was even able to plan a long trip overseas.

Tailoring the pathway to you
We developed these food strategies to provide every woman with options to create a food plan that is right for them.

Which food strategy to use?

Goal	Food strategy recommended
To support your hormones but feel you are not ready for an elimination plan	PFC
Weight control	Hormone Reset
Resolve gut issues	Microbiome Repair – if change isn't experienced within three months, move to Systemic Reset
You have tried everything and nothing has worked	Systemic Reset – full carnivore for three months followed by animal-based

Getting our diet right is key in balancing our hormones, but many people want to bypass this and get the solution in a supplement. We are huge fans of supplements, but we know that they are trying to fight a losing battle if we haven't got the right foundations in place.

We recommend finding the right food strategy first and then start looking at what you can add into your regime to support you achieve your health goals.

Supplements

In the United Kingdom, the revenue generated in the Vitamins & Minerals market reached a staggering US$0.78bn in 2024.[3] However, we see many people who are grabbing at anything they read about and are totally confused and overwhelmed.

When we were trained, there was a very gung-ho approach to supplementation, but the truth is that for people with sensitive guts and hormone issues, supplements can be very challenging to metabolize. We believe that less is more, and we teach our coaches to have a very focused strategy with supplementation.

Quality is also very important. If it cost 99p, it's either produced synthetically, which your body won't know what to do with, or full of fillers that are inflammatory.

Organic, food-state, filler-free supplementation is the way to go.

However, please do not assume that because supplements are natural, they are harmless. It is essential to check that you can take supplements with your doctor or healthcare provider, and when in doubt, work with a coach.

We work with eight types of nutritional supplementation:

- **vitamins** such as vitamin C or vitamin B that may be diminished in the body due to a poor diet or an inability to absorb

- **minerals** such as magnesium that are depleted in our food chain

- **herbs** taken for a short period of time to support endocrine or digestive function

- **digestive aids** such as digestive acid or enzymes to break down food and aid digestion

- **individual amino acids** that support specific functions throughout the body, including protein digestion, tissue repair, and nutrient absorption

- **omega 3,** which are essential fats that our body can't make

- **adaptogenic herbs** that help support the endocrine system with mitigating the impact of stress

- **other beneficial compounds.**

Let's break down what supplements are helpful for each one of our health pillars.

Supplements to support blood sugar regulation
Magnesium and zinc

Magnesium and zinc are incredibly important in the regulation of blood sugars and reducing insulin resistance. They are the "doorkeepers" that upregulate the insulin receptors of each cell and allow insulin to enter and leave. If we don't have enough magnesium or zinc, the free flow of insulin is reduced and this results in insulin resistance. According to one study in 2018, over one in ten adults (15% of males and 12% of females) had magnesium intakes below the lower reference nutrient intake (LRNI).[4]

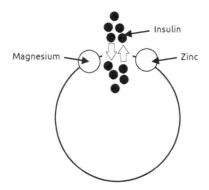

DIAGRAM 29 – THE MINERAL DOORKEEPERS OF CELLS, ZINC AND MAGNESIUM

As well as this hugely important role, they both have lots of other vital jobs.

Magnesium is the fourth most abundant mineral in the human body. It plays several important roles in more than 600 reactions in your body, including:

- energy creation – helps convert food into energy
- protein formation – helps create new proteins from amino acids
- gene maintenance – helps create and repair DNA and RNA
- muscle movements – is part of the contraction and relaxation of muscles
- nervous system regulation – helps regulate neurotransmitters, which send messages throughout your brain and nervous system.

Studies suggest that about 50 per cent of people in Europe get less than the recommended daily amount of magnesium.

All magnesium supplements will help with improving sleep, reducing anxiety, and reducing the effects of stress as well as blood sugar balancing.

The common supplement in health shops and supermarkets tends to be magnesium oxide. Magnesium oxide isn't particularly well absorbed and so is usually recommended for the relief of acute constipation.

We prefer following magnesium supplements which are all more easily absorbed than magnesium oxide and offer other benefits than just the main ones mentioned above.

- Magnesium malate is excellent for relieving muscle cramps or spasms (including period pains) and reducing fatigue. We remember it as "malate for muscles".

- Magnesium glycinate is great for people with sensitive guts. It is especially beneficial for people with loose bowels, so we remember it as "glycinate to glue up the bowels".

- Magnesium citrate is fantastic at relieving constipation but is less abrasive than magnesium oxide, so it is useful as a daily bowel support. Therefore, we remember it as "citrate for constipation".

- Magnesium taurate is known to be useful to reduce high blood pressure and to calm the nervous system. It contains the amino acid taurine which is found in energy drinks like Red Bull, as it reduces the negative effects of the high levels of caffeine in these drinks.

Finding the right magnesium is a game changer, and you can absolutely tell if it's working for you or not.

Zinc, like magnesium, is one of those incredible minerals that supports the body with so many functions, including the immune system, skin health, growth, blood sugar balancing, hormone support, and digestive function. If you are having issues within your immune function, zinc is a great supplement to choose.

Omega 3 EPA

.Omegas are essential fatty acids, and as we can't make them in the body, we need to consume them. They are brilliant for reducing inflammation and they also regulate high triglycerides.

If you are vegan and don't want to consume the omega 3 as a fish oil, it is now possible to buy omega 3 made from the algae that the fish eat, which is full of omega 3.

Omega 3 is absorbed directly into the bloodstream rather than being processed by the liver, meaning that it is a helpful fat during this hormonal transition.

Chromium

This commonly overlooked mineral is vital in blood sugar regulation as it improves our response to insulin. It is excellent for reducing sugar cravings.

Vitamin D3

This is one of the supplements that pops up for a few issues.

There is a big problem with people being vitamin D deficient either because of a lack of sunshine or because we are slapping on sun cream as soon as the sun comes out.

It acts like a hormone in the body as it stimulates insulin release while creating better insulin tolerance and improving insulin sensitivity.

Inositol

This is a type of sugar made in the body that is very helpful for weight regulation, hormone stabilization, and reducing carb addiction, but it should be avoided if you have diabetes.

Supplements to regulate stress hormones

There are many, many supplements on the market aimed at stress. We are fans of knowing what things do, so you can avoid the marketing spiel and choose a product that is right for you.

B vitamins

B vitamins support the adrenal glands and the nervous system, so are excellent if you are busy, stressed, wired, fatigued, or have a whirring brain that doesn't switch off. B vitamins also play a role in digestion.

It is also important to remember that a vegan diet and sometimes a poor vegetarian diet are lacking B vitamins, especially B12.

Those with SIBO can struggle to absorb B12, so if you have gut issues, taking a B complex can help once your SIBO is under control.

5-hydroxytryptophan (5-HTP)

This is an amino acid that your body naturally produces, and the body uses it to produce serotonin; low serotonin can lead to depression, anxiety, sleep disorders, weight gain, and other health problems. 5-HTP can cause digestive discomfort, so should be avoided with gut issues.

Co-enzyme Q10

This helps generate energy in your cells, so is useful if you have low energy or suffer with fatigue.

Inositol

Excellent for reducing anxiety and promoting sleep, it supports the production of the neurotransmitters dopamine and GABA.

Adaptogenic herbs

This is one of our favourite areas of supplementation, because when you find the right adaptogen, it can make a huge difference to your health and vitality – in a nutshell, it can change the HPA axis dysregulation that we discussed in Chapter 5.

They help by switching back on the communication from the adrenal glands to the pituitary and hypothalamus to ensure that we start producing an appropriate amount of adrenaline and cortisol.

Common symptoms that are signs you might benefit from being supported by adaptogens are fatigue and exhaustion, poor sleep, weight instability, anxiety, and digestive issues, which, by our reckoning, affect most menopausal women.

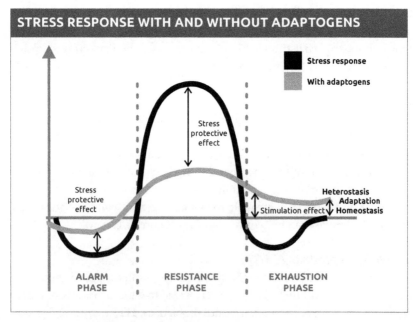

DIAGRAM 30 – THE ADAPTOGENIC STRESS RESPONSE

There are lots of different types of adaptogens, and many of them have gained a lot of press interest and are commonly known; however, it is important to find the right one for you. While they all reduce the stress response, they have other properties, which means that you can find the one that will be most beneficial.

Liquorice root
Balances blood sugars and fatigue, antiviral, stimulates digestion, reduces mucus, oestrogen-like effect (not good with oestrogen dominance), reduces hot flushes, reduces muscle cramps. *Note:* Not to be taken with high blood pressure.

Tulsi (holy basil)
Balances menopause hormones, reduces acne, supports diabetes and respiratory conditions, benefits headaches, good for eye health, reduces the effects of chemical stress.

Reishi mushroom
Reduces inflammation, fatigue, and infections; aids liver, digestion, skin, and immune function; is antiviral; balances hormones and blood sugars.

Schisandra root
Great for balancing your mental state, especially if your mind is flitting and unable to focus. Calms the adrenals, anxiety, and stress; reduces inflammation; supports the liver; increases digestive enzymes; enhances mental performance; improves sexual function; benefits the skin.

Spirulina
A fantastic nervous system support. Lowers blood pressure, reduces cholesterol, boosts energy, reduces sinus issues, supports memory. It is also a good protein source.

Panax ginseng
This is very stimulating. Improves mood, reduces stress and deep fatigue, improves brain function, anti-inflammatory, supports weight loss and blood sugar regulation.

Siberian ginseng
Enhances physical stamina and alertness, antiviral, energy boosting. Can act like an oestrogen, so be careful in perimenopause.

Rhodiola
This is used for extreme stress. It supports fat burning, is beneficial for depression, promotes energy, reduces exhaustion and fatigue, and enhances brain function.

Ashwagandha
This is very popular for use during menopause. It is excellent at reducing oestrogen dominance but also stimulates testosterone. It reduces anxiety, reduces inflammation, lowers cortisol, supports the immune system, boost stamina, enhances sleep, balances depression, supports blood sugar, boosts fertility, and lowers cholesterol.

Olive leaf
An excellent antibacterial. It boosts immune function and energy, lowers blood pressure, supports cardiovascular health and brain function, regulates gut bacteria and fungus, benefits skin, promotes wound healing, and is oestrogen balancing.

Chaste tree (Vitex agnus-castus)
Stimulates progesterone production and supports ovulation.

Gelatinized maca root
This stimulates oestrogen and progesterone, and reduces excess cortisol. It is shown to be beneficial for hot flushes and menopausal symptoms as an alternative to HRT.

Supplements for sex hormones
Oestrogen-detoxing supplements
The following three supplements are incredibly powerful and should be used with care. They are mostly beneficial during perimenopause when oestrogen dominance is causing most symptoms. They work by supporting the liver to undergo the phase 2 detoxification process more effectively.

Diindolylmethane (DIM)
DIM has three main benefits:

- metabolizes oestrogen

- frees up bound testosterone

- acts as a natural aromatase inhibitor (aromatase is an enzyme that creates more oestrogen).

N-acetyl-L-cysteine (NAC)
NAC is needed to make and replenish an important antioxidant called glutathione.

Studies show that NAC may stabilize blood sugar by decreasing inflammation in fat cells, thereby improving insulin resistance.

NAC is such an incredible supplement that its name is jokingly referred to as "Nearly All Conditions". It is used widely in pharmaceuticals as well as naturopathy.

Calcium D-glucarate

Calcium D-glucarate supports the liver to remove toxins and hormones such as oestrogen from the body. It reduces the gut's ability to reabsorb circulating oestrogen. It can also reduce harmful intestinal bacteria and has been shown to support healthy cholesterol levels.

Other supplements to balance sex hormones include:

Manganese

This is a trace mineral, which improves bone health, reduces inflammation, regulates blood sugars, helps with protein absorption, and reduces PMS symptoms in women.

Iron

Excellent for regulating light or heavy bleeding. We recommend natural iron supplements, which should not cause constipation. Often the right iron supplement can relieve constipation. The heavy bleeding itself is a sign of hormone imbalance that needs rectifying.

Soy

Soy contains plant-based chemicals called phyto-oestrogens. These chemicals act like a weaker form of oestrogen in the body. Once in your body, the soy binds to the same receptors as oestrogen and mimics their effects, which has been shown to reduce hot flushes and other symptoms of menopause.

Vitamin D3

With hormones, vitamin D regulates the production of oestrogen and progesterone, helping to keep them balanced. It is also important for maintaining bone density as this diminishes in post-menopause.

Supplements for the digestive system

There are two aspects of supplementing for the digestive system: upper digestion and bowel support.

Upper digestive support would be to manage issues such as indigestion, heartburn, bloating, and belching. Ultimately, these issues are caused by food intolerance and stress, so dealing with the underlying cause is the most important job, but that can take time. Meanwhile, digestive aids can help enormously and provide glorious relief from symptoms.

If you know what macronutrients cause your digestive symptoms, you can choose a digestive aid that has the right enzyme in it that will help with the digestion of those foods.

Digestive aid is either an enzyme, an acid, or a combination of both.

- **Amylase** breaks down carbohydrates, or starches, into sugar molecules. Insufficient amylase can lead to diarrhoea.

- **Lipase** works with bile to break down fats. If you don't have enough lipase, you'll be lacking in fat-soluble vitamins such as A, D, E, and K. If you have been on a low-fat diet for many years, you could be low in lipase production.

- **Protease** breaks down proteins into amino acids. It also helps keep bacteria and yeast under control in the intestines. A shortage of protease can lead to allergies or toxicity in the intestines.

- **Pepsin** is produced in the stomach and is one of the main digestive enzymes helping to digest proteins.

- The acid is **hydrochloric acid**. This stomach acid naturally reduces as we age. When stomach acid is low it can often lead to issues like heartburn which people often mistake for too much stomach acid. They then misguidedly try and reduce their acid when they need to increase it. To increase the production of stomach acid we can supplement with betaine hydrochloride.

To find out if you need an acid on its own or a combination, try taking ½ teaspoon of apple cider vinegar in water before you eat and see if it helps. If it doesn't help at all, go for an enzyme-only digestive aid. If it does help, it suggests acid would be helpful, so try a combination first. If that doesn't entirely diminish your symptoms, try an acid on its own.

For bowel support, there are, again, hundreds of products on the market. When we were first trained, we were taught to recommend a lot of bowel support to get bowels moving. However, our research and our own personal experience has shown that many bowels are sensitive, and we must be careful. The right magnesium and adaptogen will be a massive help and, in the case of IBS, it is commonly SIBO or gut microbiome issues. We often find that SIBO or gut microbiome issues are behind IBS and as such, we work with a carefully constructed gut microbiome protocol to *remove* any unwanted bacteria or fungus, *replace* it with the right nutrition for a happy microbiome, *reinoculate* with the right bacteria, and *repair* any damage to the intestinal lining. This can take anything from three months to a year, but it is a much more effective approach than just trying to force the bowels to move. We strongly recommend working with a coach to support you with this process.

Gut microbiome protocol

Remove with antibacterial supplements such as:

- caprylic acid

- grapefruit seed extract

- berberine (*Berberis arisata*)

- oregano extract (*Origanium vulgaris*)

- N-acetyl-L-cysteine (NAC) to remove the protective biofilm that the bacteria produces

- olive leaf (adaptogenic herb)

- diatomaceous earth – human grade (very gentle and good for parasite clearing).

Replace with:

- vitamin B12 (get a blood test from the doctor if you suspect this is low)

- fat-soluble vitamins including A, D, E, and K.

- the appropriate magnesium depending on bowel movements.

Reinoculate with prebiotics such as inulin, which creates the right environment for good bacteria to thrive.

Lactobacillus acidophilus supplements can cause digestive issues, so instead try soil-based probiotics or *Saccharomyces boulardii*, but if that still causes problems, go for a more inert form of probiotic such as terrahydrite, a mineral supplement that comes from the soil, or try eating more fermented foods such as sauerkraut and kombucha (these can exacerbate SIBO; if symptoms occur, revisit the remove phase).

Repair with:

- L-glutamine
- L-arginine
- zinc

- omega 3
- deglycyrrhizinated licorice
- collagen and bone broth.

Supplements for the immune system

Because the immune system is a victim of an imbalanced triangle, we want to make sure that the three main pillars are in place first. If working on blood sugars, stress, and hormone balancing isn't enough, then look at immune supplementation.

The focus with the immune system is helping your body to manage inflammation and supporting your immune system with essential nutrients so it can do its job effectively. As you will see from the list of essential nutrients below, many of these nutrients are relevant to other aspects of the triangle, so you will be getting cross-referenced benefits.

- Antioxidants vitamins including A, C, D, and E.

- Anti-inflammatory adaptogens including reishi mushroom.

- L-arginine and L-glutamine for reducing inflammation through gut repair.

- Zinc for immune support.

- Omega 3 for its anti-inflammatory properties.

- NAC is a powerful antioxidant, ridding the body of cell-damaging free radicals and supporting the body to detox. It is also anti-inflammatory.

- Selenium boosts white blood cells and supports fighting infection.

- Inositol promotes T cell immunity regulation and has anti-inflammatory properties.

It's still a minefield – where do I start?

We recommend that if you want to try supplementing and have no health issues that are contraindicated, you start with a core selection of:

- the right magnesium

- an adaptogen that best fits your health profile

- vitamin D3 or Omega 3.

Then choose the priority area you need to focus on, such as:

- a digestive enzyme to help you break down food, reduce heartburn or indigestion, and absorb properly

- SIBO supplementation (as described in the gut microbiome protocol on the previous page)

- an oestrogen-detoxing supplement

- immune support.

But we don't recommend doing it all at once unless you've been advised by a coach. Balance the Triangle of Hormonal Health and make sure you can digest properly, take the supplements for a month, and then reassess.

How often do I take them?
Follow the supplement recommendations on the pot. If a supplement recommends 1–3 tablets per day, for example, start low with one tablet a day, and increase the following week if needed.

Diet and mindset
Mindset is important when we are changing diet and lifestyle habits. The way you think about these changes will completely affect the outcome.

Some people can throw themselves into a new regime easily, whereas others need to spend time planning, getting their head into it, and getting some support.

The important thing is to know what you need to be successful.

Spending some time reflecting on your beliefs and behaviours around food can be impactful in making sure you reach your goals.

Do you believe that you need a quick fix or a fad diet that is going to transform the way you feel and look? If yes, this could use some reframing to shift your mindset from wanting a quick fix to wanting a permanent lifestyle change.

Are you worried that you will be too restricted and eating like this is a punishment? If so, working with a coach can help you create sustainable change and learn some emotional tools to keep you motivated.

Here are a few tips we've learned along the way.

#1 Stop the guilt
If you slip up, please don't punish or criticize yourself. Be gentle with yourself, observe why you made the choices you made, and learn from them, and then just pick up where you left off.

#2 Think about what you can have, not what you can't
Thinking about the food you can't eat just creates a sense of lack and misery.

If you are committing to quitting wheat, for example, focus on the abundance of wonderful fresh meals you can enjoy made with meat, fish, fruit, and vegetables, rather than the boring sandwich you can't have.

#3 Healthy eating is a form of self-care

Healthy eating and exercise are two important forms of self-care, so we need to reframe how we think about them. Focus on healthy foods you enjoy and think about how much this food is nourishing you and supporting your hormones. Note the change in how you're feeling when you are eating well and how your symptoms have changed. These changes are the ultimate reward!

#4 Be realistic

One of the reasons we have a staged approach with our food strategies is because not everyone can commit to a strict elimination plan. Radically changing everything may prove to be too overwhelming, and it may set you up for disappointment, so assess where you are now and what feels right for you. It is better to make one small sustainable change every week and succeed, rather than trying to do too much, too quickly, and giving in.

#5 Ditch the willpower

The existence of willpower is a huge con, and believing in it means we are setting ourselves up to a version of the world where we aren't good enough if we don't achieve perfection.

Instead of talking about willpower, we talk about desire and discipline. These are the two traits we need to succeed.

Desire is the key to setting realistic goals. Do we *really* want what we think we want? Do we want it enough to make changes that can feel tough? If the answer is no, then be honest with yourself about it rather than going around in circles. But if the answer is yes, then we need to discuss discipline.

Discipline isn't something we are born with; it's something we learn. And there are tools and tricks and hacks to help us become successful. How can you beat yourself up for not being good at something if you haven't learned the skills?

This is why we are fans of working with a coach. They will help you learn the tools and hold you accountable.

If your discipline is in place but you aren't feeling it, check back in on that desire.

#6 Get help if you need it

If you know you struggle with committing to yourself and you have many years of poor eating habits to unlearn, choose to work with a coach who can help you work through these issues.

Food addiction

We want to talk a bit about food addiction. Currently, food addiction hasn't got an official medical classification, but thousands of coaches and doctors working with clients are all too aware that this addiction is real and is a form of eating disorder.

We believe it is caused in part by the foods we are choosing, in part by the marketing spin food is given, and in part as a response to the amount of stress that people are facing today.

If you struggle with food addiction, or any eating disorder, please work with a trained coach or doctor. We have added some great places to seek support in the resources in Chapter 16.

Living your life

Reading this book may have inspired you to commit to a food plan for, say, three months, and you might be wondering where to fit it into your schedule so you can stay at home and manage all your own meals. Alternatively, you might be thinking that you can't commit to any of the food strategies because you can't fit them into your life. However, these plans are designed to be applied to your everyday life and that means navigating restaurants, travelling, holidays, birthday parties, and family meals.

Sharing food and meals is a central part of the human experience.

The feedback we commonly hear is that once people have embedded the changes to their diets, they are able to navigate any situation. But let's also remember that there is no "fail". Choosing to eat something off plan won't be the end of the world; we just get back on the plan when we can.

Whichever food strategy you are working with, it can be useful to know that the PFC approach to eating is a fallback when all else fails. This way, you won't overload on sugar or carbohydrates that will destabilize your blood sugars, and it will keep the foundations in place. For example, if you are eating out and want to drink alcohol, load up on the protein and fats, and choose the booze as your carb option.

Choose your indulgences wisely and have something you are really going to love. Eat it mindfully with lots of enjoyment and zero guilt. And if you want that glass of wine or piece of birthday cake, ensure you support it with a protein and fat food choice alongside.

Practise saying "no thank you". Most people offer you food because they want to be kind and show their love. Thanking them and saying no is usually enough.

Become mindful of your individual triggers. You might be able to get away with a glass of wine at a party without any symptoms reappearing, but not eating a sandwich without suffering for it later. Learn what your body is telling you and make the food choices accordingly. Treats stop feeling like treats when they instantly give us agonizing headaches or digestive pain.

TAKE-HOME MESSAGE

Find the food strategy that works for you and choose targeted supplementation that most suits where you are in your health journey. If you need help with your mindset, work with a coach who can support you!

— CHAPTER 15 —

Conclusion

Too many women accept feeling unwell during the menopause transition as the "norm".

It doesn't have to be, and we don't have to resign ourselves to a life of not feeling brilliant, but HRT on its own will not be the magic bullet.

By getting our health foundations in place, ensuring we are absorbing properly, have removed obvious stressors, and have found the right food strategy to support our gut and hormones, we are giving our HRT or the natural options a chance to help us feel amazing.

A challenging menopause doesn't come out of the blue and can be traced back to issues that have been going on, often under the radar, for years – IBS, migraines, and period issues are all potential signs that our Triangle of Hormonal Health needs some work.

If we were to summarize the entirety of this book, we would say that the key to improving the menopause experience is to undertake a "whole-health" approach:

- Increase your protein intake (a dedicated protein source at every meal) and reduce your carbohydrate load to support blood sugar stabilization and to ensure a nutrient-dense diet.

- Remove wheat, dairy, and sugar from your diet and reduce processed food.

- If you still have symptoms, use the food intolerance hierarchy to work out which foods you are intolerant to and remove them from your diet.

- Drink enough water and avoid too much alcohol and caffeine.

- Work on all aspects of stress to reduce cortisol.

- Speak to your doctor about swapping synthetic progesterone for body-identical progesterone (with oestrogen). Synthetic hormones will not help you. Keep pushing back if your doctor is resistant to this swap. If you still don't feel brilliant after making the swap, seek support from a menopause coach.

- Clean up your gut to ensure you can metabolize oestrogen.

- Do the right exercise at the right time of day.

- Remove the toxic chemicals from your life and avoid xeno-oestrogens.

- Focus on your sleep hygiene and rest when you need to.

- Find some supplements to support you.

- Find some tools or a coach to help you work through your emotions. It's time to leave your baggage behind and work on emotional resilience and boundaries.

- Develop a self-love and gratitude practice.

- Prioritize getting out into nature!

- Remember, you can't do all this overnight. Make one change at a time, work out which items in the list are most impactive, and then keep doing them. Step by step, one day at a time…

- And, most importantly, on the bad days, remember that "this too shall pass".

We hope that this book means you can have a smoother menopause transition. But we also wish for you that it is transformative and allows you to fiercely grab the next phase of your life so that you can live it radically.

With much love and blessings.

— CHAPTER 16 —

Next steps and resources

We really hope that this book has inspired you to take the next step in supporting your own health or the health of women you are working with. If you have found this useful, please spread the word about our work.

Below are some suggestions for the next steps on the path.

Become a coach!

The world is full of women who are determined to feel better and who are drowning in conflicting information and not being supported by the doctors. There is a desperate, desperate need for more well-trained coaches.

If you are interested in learning more about this work and becoming a menopause or wellness coach, or to look at some of the talks we've done on hormones, visit www.functional-wellness.co.uk to explore more about our internationally accredited training programmes.

We have hundreds of free videos available on our YouTube channel @functionalwellnesscollege (please subscribe to the channel if you find the information useful!), and our social media channels are also full of information.

For your health

If you are interested in the foundations of health but aren't sure where to start or which food strategy you should be looking at, you can take our free online assessment (www.hormone-wellness.co.uk/symptom-assessor) which will give you an option to purchase an online toolkit to work with our food strategies along with lifestyle and supplement suggestions. We also have lots of free information on this website including podcasts and blogs to support you.

You can also find details of our food strategies, recipes, and useful tools such as a downloadable hormone tracker on our website (www.hormone-wellness.co.uk/product/hormone-tracker).

For your emotions

Check out our online emotional programme Reclaim Your Life on our website (www.hormone-wellness.co.uk/reclaim-your-life-online).

Choosing a wellness or menopause coach

You may choose to work with a health or menopause coach to help you navigate your wellness journey. A qualified coach can be knowledgeable and experienced, and will be able to tailor a process like ours for your needs and help you troubleshoot any obstacles you experience. It can also be very empowering to talk to someone about how you're feeling, both emotionally and physically.

To support women in their quest for good health and coaching they can trust, we created an online clinic offering. Our coaches are all highly trained and experienced in our methods and will work with you to create the right pathway for your needs and goals. For more information, visit www.hormone-wellness.co.uk. We have also trained hundreds of menopause coaches and functional kinesiologists who work with the Triangle of Hormonal Health and the food strategies (plus kinesiologists are excellent at food sensitivity testing and have a myriad of other amazing tools and techniques at their disposal). Details of our practitioners are on our college websites listed below.

If you choose to go to elsewhere, here are our top tips for choosing a health coach.

- Ensure that the health coach you work with is qualified and experienced. Look for certifications and credentials that demonstrate their expertise in the field. Watch out for coaches who only have short-course certificates.

- Make sure your coach has a governing body and insurance.

- A good health coach will have a holistic understanding of women's health, including hormones, nutrition, food, lifestyle, and natural options of HRT.

- Your chosen coach may offer individual coaching sessions, group workshops, or a combination of both. Discuss the various methods available and decide what works best for you.

- A good coach will be able to order laboratory tests to do deeper investigation on areas such as gut health and function and hormone function tests (DUTCH test).

Visiting the doctor

In our experience, women can be ignored, fobbed off, or gaslit when approaching the medical profession with hormonal or menopausal issues.

If you would like a letter to print to take to the GP to support you with your requests for body-identical hormones, please visit www.hormone-wellness.co.uk/Dear-GP.

Here are some key areas to ensure that your appointment with your GP better meets your needs:

- Plan. Write down any symptoms or questions you have.

- Most of us only have 12 minutes with our GP, so it's crucial for you to make that time count. Before your appointment, write down anything about your body that may seem off or different. This way, you are getting your questions answered and focusing your GP to engage in what you are saying.

- Be honest about what is going on.

- Don't hide anything, regardless of your embarrassment, as it may affect your treatment options. Examples include drug taking, smoking, or sexual activity. Your doctor really does need this information to provide you with the best possible care, screenings, and treatment.

- Be clear about what you want and what you don't want.

- Do not be fobbed off with the pill or the Mirena coil. Be clear that you do not want synthetic hormones and you want to explore body-identical alternatives. This is your health, you are in charge of it, and it is your doctor's role to work with you and ensure that a pathway is medically viable based on your health history, not dictate what happens.

- You are entitled to judgement-free healthcare where are you not challenged or questioned on why you may want something like Utrogestan.

Know your rights.

As a patient some of your key rights are to:

- receive NHS services free of charge

- not be discriminated against

- be treated with professional standards by qualified and experienced staff

- expect NHS organizations to monitor and try to improve continuously the quality of their services

- be treated with dignity and respect

- accept or refuse treatment and only be physically examined with consent

- be given information about any test and treatment options open to you, what they involve, and their risks and benefits

- have access to your own records

- privacy and confidentiality

- have any complaint acknowledged within three days and properly investigated

- compensation if harmed by negligent treatment.

Remember, it's OK to ask to see another doctor if you're not happy.

This is your health, and you are entitled to a doctor who respects you, listens to you, and empowers you to do better when you leave their office. Request a second appointment if you are not happy with the outcome.

Resources

The following are resources that we have found to be very beneficial on the menopause journey:

For more information on low-carb diets, check out the Public Health Collaboration (https://phcuk.org), and for the animal-based approach Dr Paul Saladino (www.paulsaladinomd.co), Dr Anthony Chafee (www.instagram.com/anthonychaffeemd), and Dr Kevin Stocks (www.kevinstock.io).

If you are struggling with standard HRT or are having a challenging menopause, some women benefit from a bespoke compounded approach. Please contact us at info@hormone-wellness.co.uk for more information.

To reclaim your sexiness through the perimenopause to post-menopause transition, we recommend a great online programme by the fantastic Dr Claire Macauley (www.pleasurepossibility.com) for women who want deeper intimacy, body confidence, and great sex.

There is a fantastic website – www.menopause.co.uk – which is full of expert advice from coaches and doctors to help support you to make decisions that feel right for your menopause transition.

Women often ask for specific exercise for hormone balancing, and we adore the work of Abi Adams at Project Woman (www.abiadams.co.uk).

On social media, it's worth looking at the work of Lara Briden (www.larabriden.com) and Nicole Jardim (www.nicolejardim.com) – and, of course, OURS! Our details are at the end of this chapter.

We also strongly recommend the book *Unwell Women* by Elinor Cleghorn if you want to understand how poorly women's health has been dealt with for millennia.

There are now menopause groups popping up all over the place in local communities and online. These groups of supportive women are getting together to share information and help each other through the menopause process, and it's inspirational to see. This is how women have always created revolution. Check out social media for your local group.

Please get in touch with us on social media or at our websites and join our fight to change the way women's hormonal health is currently dealt with.

- www.hormone-wellness.co.uk

- www.functional-wellness.co.uk; FB: @functionalwellnesscourses; IG: @functionalwellnessofficial; YouTube channel: @functional wellnesscollege

- www.functionalkinesiology.co.uk; FB: @functionalkinesiology courses; IG: @functionalkinesiologyuk

- www.clairesnowdon-darling.com; FB, TikTok and IG @clairesnow-dondarlingofficial

Claire is delighted to be the menopause advisor for The Dawn Treaders. A three-woman ocean rowing team – Annabel, Kat, and Nicole – will be attempting to row across the Pacific Ocean from California to Hawaii, starting in June 2028.

These three women will be in their mid- to late 40s when doing this row. They want to use the project to share their journey, not only across the ocean but through perimenopause, to help empower and educate other women to remind them that they are capable of far more than they imagined.

Find out more at www.dawntreaders.ro

— CHAPTER 17 —

Frequently Asked Questions

Should I start hormone therapy?

This is a question unique to all women, and it deserves time, research, and consideration to find the right solution. It really depends on how badly your life is affected by symptoms. If you've sailed through menopause, you might not feel the need to use HRT, but if you are struggling, it could be worthwhile. Speak to a coach and your GP to get all the information you need to make an informed decision.

How will the menopause affect my sex drive?

As hormones fluctuate through perimenopause and menopause, your sex drive may also change. In perimenopause, the lowering of progesterone and testosterone and the fluctuating oestrogen can lower desire and make it more difficult to become aroused. At menopause and beyond, the loss of oestrogen further compounds the issue.

Will nutritional supplements treat my symptoms?

Nutritional supplements can be incredibly supportive for your health and menopausal journey, but they are not going to "treat" your symptoms. View supplements as a support to your wellness rather than a solution to symptoms.

My HRT is not working; what do I do?

There are three main areas we would be looking at if HRT is causing you issues. Number one: you could be on the wrong type of HRT or dosage. Number two: the foundations of your wellness are not in place, such as diet and lifestyle factors, and they need addressing. Number three: if you are taking your HRT orally, you may not be absorbing correctly, so supporting your digestive system may help.

I haven't had a period in a year; am I menopausal?

Yes, you are considered menopausal. Please note that you may have the occasional bleed after 12 months of no menstrual cycles.

How do I know if I am menopausal?

Officially, a woman who is in menopause is a woman who has not had a menstrual cycle in 12 months. If you are experiencing hormone changes like hot flushes, but are still experiencing periods, no matter how irregular, you are considered perimenopausal.

I'm on the Mirena coil: what should I do?

Mirena is a synthetic progestin-releasing IUD and considered a medication and HRT treatment; therefore, we are unable to make recommendations or give advice in this area. However, we recommend that you revisit Chapter 6 on sex hormones and decide whether removing the Mirena coil feels right for you. If you make the decision to remove the device, you are within your rights to request this from your doctor.

I'm on the pill: what should I do?

Like the Mirena coil answer above, the contraceptive pill is a medication and HRT treatment, and we are unable to make recommendations or give advice in this area. However, we recommend that you revisit Chapter 6 on sex hormones and decide whether discontinuing the contraceptive pill feels right for you.

How do I know if I'm in perimenopause?

Traditionally, symptoms of perimenopause included hot flushes or changes in menstrual cycles. However, we are seeing women with symptoms such as insomnia, headaches, and weight gain as part of perimenopause with no changes in their cycles.

If you want to test for perimenopause, there are a few ways to do this. If you are under 40, and in the UK, the NHS will take two blood tests six weeks apart to measure levels of follicle-stimulating hormone (FSH). High levels of FSH may indicate perimenopause.

If you would like to test privately, you can work with a menopause coach who can order a Dried Urine Test for Comprehensive Hormones (DUTCH test), which measures adrenal and sex hormones over a 24-hour timeframe, five days after ovulation.

My doctor has recommended a hysterectomy; what do I do?

A hysterectomy is a big decision for any woman and needs consideration, research, and some direct questions with your surgeon, including "Is this surgery necessary?" and "Are there other options?"

There are some instances where a hysterectomy is the best solution – for example, cancer of the womb, ovaries, or cervix. However, in cases of heavy periods or pelvic pain, there are options that may support your health enough not to need a hysterectomy, and so the question for your surgeon could be "Can I have six months to work on this issue?"

I've had a hysterectomy; can I have body-identical progesterone?

Yes, but most doctors say no, so keep asking for a second opinion until you find one who understands this!

How long until I see results of the food and lifestyle recommendations?

Everyone is unique. Some women experience improvement in a matter of days. Other women take longer. If you have been struggling with your health for years, allow time for change to happen. It can be frustrating, and we often want immediate results, but health can be a journey and an unfolding that takes time.

I don't want to stop being a vegan; what should I eat?

To support your body, ensure you are supplementing to replace the nutrients you are missing and include protein sources such as protein powder, tofu, and soya to ensure you are eating PFC.

I have recovered from breast cancer which put me in early menopause; how do I manage my hormones?

The best way to manage your hormonal health is to follow the wellness guidelines and strategies in this book. With regard to HRT, read Chapter

How can I check my hormones?

If you want to test for perimenopause, there are a few ways to do this. If you are under 40, the NHS in the UK will take two blood tests six weeks apart to measure levels of follicle-stimulating hormone (FSH). High levels of FSH may indicate perimenopause. They don't test for progesterone, which means that you won't get the full picture.

If you would like to test privately, you can work with a menopause coach who can order a Dried Urine Test for Comprehensive Hormones (DUTCH test), which measures adrenal and sex hormones over a 24-hour timeframe, five days after ovulation.

I am ten years post-menopause; is it too late for HRT?

The low-dose natural HRT options, including herbal remedies, are likely to be ineffective. You can speak to your GP about the possibility of taking prescribed HRT and the options available to you.

I have menosomnia – help!

It's awful, isn't it? We recommend following the guidelines in this book around sleep hygiene in Chapter 11 and speaking to your GP about HRT including progesterone, which is important for sleep.

How long should I be on HRT?

There's no fixed limit on how long you can take HRT. Evidence from a Cochrane data-analysis as well as long-term data from the Women's Health Initiative showed no increase in cardiovascular issues or all-cause mortality in women who initiated HRT more than ten years after menopause.[1]

What birth control do you recommend?

We recommend condoms, the copper IUD, natural family planning, and, if you are in a long-term relationship, to discuss the option of a vasectomy for your partner.

I have a thyroid imbalance; should I be doing something different?

As the thyroid gland is part of your endocrine system and produces hormones that have a direct effect on your ovaries and sexual organs, having a thyroid imbalance will affect and could worsen your perimenopause and menopause experience. We recommend exploring ways to support your thyroid, be it with medication (consulting with your doctor), dietary (avoid goitrogenic foods such as raw brassicas), or taking iodine supplements (not recommended for autoimmune thyroid conditions).

I have hormone imbalance, gut problems, and heightened immune responses; which strategy is best for me?

These issues can often go together, so please know that you are not alone. We would recommend starting with the PFC Food Strategy and once you are comfortable with this (within 1–3 months), move to the Microbiome Food Repair Strategy. If you are not experiencing the results you are looking for after six months, move to the Systemic Reset Food Strategy. Partnered with your food plan, adopt the healthy lifestyle practices including stress relief, movement of your body, and sleep hygiene (Chapter 11).

I've got the Mirena coil; can I have natural progesterone?

The answer should be no, but we have seen many clients who have both.

What are the signs that my HRT is not working?

If you are experiencing menopausal symptoms after several months on HRT, it is likely something needs reviewing and changing. It is advised that it takes several weeks to feel the benefit and up to three months before the effects are fully realized.

Is there a risk of increased breast cancer with women on HRT?

The NHS state that the risk is low and that there are approximately five extra cases of breast cancer in every 1000 women who take combined HRT for five years.[2] The risk increases the longer you take it and the older you are.

However, these studies don't differentiate between women on synthetic hormones and body-identical hormones, and we don't have this data available.

However, the drop in hormones through menopause can also cause cancer, stroke, and osteoporosis, so both decisions – to take HRT or not to take it – carry risk.

I am experiencing weight gain on HRT; what can I do?

Weight gain is listed as a potential side effect of taking HRT. Imbalanced oestrogen levels (either too high or too low) can contribute to weight gain and fluctuations because oestrogen plays a role in metabolism and insulin resistance, which affect appetite, energy levels, and body fat storage. The synthetic form of progesterone, progestin, acts as a stimulator rather than a calmer, which increases stress and metabolic dysfunction. If you are gaining weight on your HRT, it is recommended to explore changing the type of HRT or dosage.

I experience breast pain on HRT; is this common?

Yes, and if it doesn't settle down within a few months, it could be that your HRT isn't working for you, or you are on the wrong dose of oestrogen. Go back to your doctor and ask them to review it.

Can I take HRT for migraines?

Fluctuations in hormones through perimenopause can bring on migraines and headaches, and the correct type and dose of HRT can relieve these symptoms. However, some HRT can contribute to headaches and migraines, so it is important to speak with a medical professional to find the best HRT for you.

Thanks and acknowledgements

Thanks to Carole McMurray for ensuring this book happened and the fantastic team at Jessica Kingsley Publishers. Having a deadline really spurred us on!

Thanks to Abi Adams of Project Woman for her exercise advice, Kate Hicks for sorting the referencing (we could not have done it without you), and Chantelle Duncan, as always, for making our work so beautiful.

We are so grateful to our fantastic faculty who are spreading the word and training excellent clinicians to help change the world one woman at a time. Thanks to our students and practitioners who have heard the call to be part of the change and to our patient "behind the scenes" team who support us to do this work.

To N and the clients who inspired the Triangle of Hormonal Health – thank you for helping us see what was really going on.

Thank you to every single client and woman who trusted us with your health and your stories. This work wouldn't have happened without you, and we are humbled and grateful to have been part of your journey. To the menopause groups that have invited us to speak – your groups are how revolutions start. Please keep up the good work.

Claire would like to thank:

Mya Rose Florrie – You are the reason for this work and my constant endeavour to make the world a better place. My deepest hope is that my work means you don't have to fight as hard as I've had to. I am deeply proud of you and of our journey. I love you with every fibre of my being.

Karl – Thank you for your support, your patience, your humour, your daily challenging, and your perspective. I adore you, darling.

BM – You have helped me more than you will ever know. Having someone who understands this process has been invaluable. "Do your best."

Laura – Whoever thought that we would end up doing what we are doing? This has been a wild ride and there's no one else I would rather be sitting next to. Let's keep going, Thelma...

Laura would like to thank:

Matthew – Thank you for believing in me. Your brilliant mind helps me explore complicated topics and uncover new insights. You hold my work to a higher standard, and you challenge me to question everything. Thank you, darling.

My parents – For supporting me in the beginning to jack in a corporate career and pursue my heart's desire. And thank you for instilling a ridiculously strong work ethic in me. It's paid off.

Claire – Thanks for being a sacrificial hormonal lamb. If it wasn't for your determination and courage to understand and overcome your own challenging menopause, we wouldn't have developed this work together. You pave the path and continue to do so, making it less bumpy for the rest of us.

References

Chapter 1

1 National Institutes of Health (n.d.) History of women's participation in clinical research. https://orwh.od.nih.gov/toolkit/recruitment/history
2 Abbasi, K. (2023) Under-representation of women in research: A status quo that is a scandal. *BMJ 2023*, 382, 2091. www.bmj.com/content/bmj/382/bmj.p2091.full.pdf
3 Hewings-Martin, Y. and Giodano, F. (2004) Diet may counteract menopause metabolism change, ZOE study shows. ZOE. https://zoe.com/learn/menopause-metabolism-study

Chapter 2

1 Office for National Statistics (2024) Suicides in England and Wales: 2023 registrations. www.ons.gov.uk/peoplepopulationandcommunity/birthsdeathsandmarriages/deaths/bulletins/suicidesintheunitedkingdom/2023
2 Australian Government (2024) *Deaths by suicide over time*. https://www.aihw.gov.au/suicide-self-harm-monitoring/data/deaths-by-suicide-in-australia/suicide-deaths-over-time
3 Vankar, Preeti (2024) *Female suicide rate in the U.S.* from 2001 to 2021, by age group. https://www.statista.com/statistics/1114127/female-suicide-rate-in-the-us-by-age-group
4 NHS England and NHS Improvement (2022) *Why is the menopause relevant to our organisation and to me and my team?* https://www.england.nhs.uk/midlands/wp-content/uploads/sites/46/2022/01/NHSEI-Menopause-Awareness-Training-Pack-v4-.pdf
5 Davis, S.R., Taylor, S., Hemachandra, C., Magraith, K. *et al.* (2023) The 2023 Practitioner's Toolkit for Managing Menopause. *Climacteric 26*, 6, 517–536. https://doi.org/10.1080/13697137.2023.2258783

Chapter 4

1 Simpson, S.J. and Raubenheimer, D. (2005) Obesity: The protein leverage hypothesis. *Obesity Reviews 6*, 2, 133–142. https://doi.org/10.1111/j.1467-789x.2005.00178.x
2 Salmerón, J., Manson, J.E., Stampfer, M.J., Colditz, G.A., Wing, A.L., and Willett, W.C. (1997) Dietary fiber, glycemic load, and risk of non-insulin-dependent diabetes mellitus in women. *JAMA 277*, 6, 472–477. https://doi.org/10.1001/jama.1997.03540300040031

Chapter 5

1 Mental Health Foundation (2018) Stressed nation: 74% of UK "overwhelmed or unable to cope" at some point in the past year. www.mentalhealth.org.uk/about-us/news/survey-stressed-nation-UK-overwhelmed-unable-to-cope
2 World Health Organization (2023) Stress. www.who.int/news-room/questions-and-answers/item/stress
3 Pappas, S. (2009) Good stress response enhances recovery from surgery, Stanford study shows. Stanford Medicine News Center. https://med.stanford.edu/news/all-news/2009/12/good-stress-response-enhances-recovery-from-surgery-stanford-study-shows.html

Chapter 6

1 Li, Y., Adur, M.K., Kannan, A., Davila, J. *et al.* (2016) Progesterone alleviates endometriosis via inhibition of uterine cell proliferation, inflammation and angiogenesis in an immunocompetent mouse model. *PLOS ONE 11*, 10, e0165347. https://doi.org/10.1371/journal.pone.0165347. This study showed that natural progesterone was effective in rats, but it was a small study.
2 Lee, J., Han, Y., Cho, H.H., and Kim, M.-R. (2019) Sleep disorders and menopause. *Journal of Menopausal Medicine 2019*, 25, 83–87. https://e-jmm.org/pdf/10.6118/jmm.19192
3 Lee, J.R. and Hopkins, V. (2003) *What Your Doctor May Not Tell You About Menopause: The Breakthrough Book on Natural Progesterone.* Warner Books.

Chapter 7

1 Svensson, A., Brunkwall, L., Roth, B., Orho-Melander, M., and Ohlsson, B. (2021) Associations between endometriosis and gut microbiota. *Reproductive Sciences 28*, 2367–2377. https://doi.org/10.1007/s43032-021-00506-5; Talwar, C., Singh, V., and Kommagani, R. (2022) The gut microbiota: A double-edged sword in endometriosis. *Biology of Reproduction 107*, 4, 881–901. https://doi.org/10.1093%2Fbiolre%2Fioac147
2 Porges, S.W. (2001) The polyvagal theory: Phylogenetic substrates of a social nervous system. *International Journal of Psychophysiology 42*, 2, 123–146. www.wisebrain.org/Polyvagal_Theory.pdf

Chapter 8

1 Keestra, S.M., Male, V., and Salai, G.D. (2021) Out of balance: The role of evolutionary mismatches in sex disparity in autoimmune disease. *Medical Hypotheses 151*, 110558. https://doi.org/10.1016/j.mehy.2021.110558
2 Straub, R.H. (2007) 'The Complex Role of Estrogens in Inflammation', *Endocrine Reviews*, 28, 5, 521–574, https://doi.org/10.1210/er.2007-0001

Chapter 11

1   NB. Eggs are listed separately as they are incorrectly considered to be dairy but they don't come from a cow or produced from milk.
2   Diamanti-Kandarakis, E., Bourguignon, J.P., Giudice, L.C., Hauser, R. *et al.* (2009) Endocrine-disrupting chemicals: An Endocrine Society scientific statement. *Endocrine Reviews 30*, 4, 293–342. https://doi.org/10.1210/er.2009-0002
3   Cited in Malkan, S. (2007) *Not Just a Pretty Face: The Ugly Side of the Beauty Industry.* New Society Publishers.
4   Cited in Malkan, S. (2007) *Not Just a Pretty Face: The Ugly Side of the Beauty Industry.* New Society Publishers.
5   Centers for Disease Control and Prevention (2016) 1 in 3 adults don't get enough sleep [Press Release]. https://archive.cdc.gov/www_cdc_gov/media/releases/2016/p0215-enough-sleep.html
6   International Agency for Research on Cancer (2011) IARC classifies radiofrequency electromagnetic fields as possibly carcinogenic to humans [Press Release]. www.iarc.who.int/wp-content/uploads/2018/07/pr208_E.pdf
7   Schertz, K.E. and Berman, M.G. (2019) Understanding nature and its cognitive benefits. *International Journal of Social Psychology 28*, 5. https://doi.org/10.1177/0963721419854100
8   British Heart Foundation (2023) 7 ways to reduce your stress by enjoying nature. www.bhf.org.uk/informationsupport/heart-matters-magazine/wellbeing/ways-to-reduce-stress-by-enjoying-nature

Chapter 12

1   Mayor, S. (2002) Review warns that risks of long term HRT outweigh benefits. *BMJ 325*, 7366, 673. https://pmc.ncbi.nlm.nih.gov/articles/PMC1124208
2   Lundberg, G., Wu, P., and Wenger, N. (2020) Menopausal hormone therapy: A comprehensive review. *Current Atherosclerosis Reports 22*, 33. https://doi.org/10.1007/s11883-020-00854-8
3   Fleischman, D.S., Navarrete, C.D., and Fessler, D.M.T. (2010) Oral contraceptives suppress ovarian hormone production. *Psychological Science 21*, 5, 750–752. https://doi.org/10.1177/0956797610368062
4   Food and Drug Administration (2008) Mirena® (levonorgestrel-releasing intrauterine system). www.accessdata.fda.gov/drugsatfda_docs/label/2008/021225s019lbl.pdf
5   Writing Group for the Women's Health Initiative Investigators (2002) Risks and benefits of estrogen plus progestin in healthy postmenopausal women: Principal results from the Women's Health Initiative randomized controlled trial. *JAMA 288*, 4, 321–333. https://doi.org/10.1001/jama.288.3.321
6   Prior, J.C. (2018) Progesterone for treatment of symptomatic menopausal women. *Climacteric 21*, 4, 358–365. www.tandfonline.com/doi/epdf/10.1080/13697137.2018.1472567?src=getftr
7   Women in Balance Institute (2024) Progesterone and bone health: Research summary. https://womeninbalance.org/resources-research/progesterone-bone-health
8   Valentino, R., Savastano, S., Tommaselli, A.P., Riccio, A. *et al.* (1993) Hormonal pattern in women affected by rheumatoid arthritis. *Journal of Endocrinological Investigation 16*, 8, 619–624. https://doi.org/10.1007/bf03347683

9 Calman, B. (2023) Celebrity menopause doctor who campaigns with Davina McCall and Mariella Frostrup accused of putting women at risk of cancer by prescribing "alarmingly high" doses of HRT. MailOnline. www.dailymail.co.uk/health/article-11927783/Is-Britains-foremost-menopause-doctor-risking-womens-lives-alarmingly-high-doses-HRT.html; British Menopause Society (2022) BMS Statement – HRT prescribing. https://thebms.org.uk/2022/12/bms-statement-hrt-prescribing

Chapter 13

1 Barański, M., Średnicka-Tober, D., Volakakis, N., Seal, C. *et al.* (2014) Higher antioxidant and lower cadmium concentrations and lower incidence of pesticide residues in organically grown crops: A systematic literature review and meta-analyses. *British Journal of Nutrition 112*, 5, 794–811. https://doi.org/10.1017/s0007114514001366

2 Średnicka-Tober, D., Barański, M., Seal, C., Sanderson, R. *et al.* (2016) Composition differences between organic and conventional meat: A systematic literature review and meta-analysis. *British Journal of Nutrition 115*, 6, 994–1011. https://doi.org/10.1017/s0007114515005073

3 Environmental Working Group (2024) The 2024 Dirty Dozen™. www.ewg.org/foodnews/dirty-dozen.php

4 Environmental Working Group (2024) The 2024 Clean Fifteen™. www.ewg.org/foodnews/clean-fifteen.php

5 Getting, J.E., Gregoire, J.R., Phul, A., and Kasten, M.J. (2013) Oxalate nephropathy due to "juicing": Case report and review. *American Journal of Medicine 126*, 9, 768–772. https://doi.org/10.1016/j.amjmed.2013.03.019; Makkapati, S., D'Agati, V.D. and Balsam, L. (2018) "Green smoothie cleanse" causing acute oxalate nephropathy. *American Journal of Kidney Diseases 71*, 2, 281–286. https://doi.org/10.1053/j.ajkd.2017.08.002

6 www.sacredcow.info

Chapter 14

1 Dr Ede's website: www.diagnosisdiet.com

2 Dr Clemens' website: www.paleomedicina.com/en/dr-zsofia-clemens

3 Statista Market Insights (2024) *Vitamins & Minerals - United Kingdom*. https://www.statista.com/outlook/hmo/otc-pharmaceuticals/vitamins-minerals/united-kingdom

4 Derbyshire, E. (2018) Micronutrient intakes of British adults across mid-life: A secondary analysis of the UK National Diet and Nutrition Survey. *Frontiers in Nutrition 5*, 55. https://doi.org/10.3389/fnut.2018.00055

Chapter 17

1 Cited in Hamoda, H., Panay, N., Pedder, H., Arya, R., and Savvas, M. (2021) BMS and WHC's 2020 recommendations on hormone replacement therapy in menopausal women. British Menopause Society. https://thebms.org.uk/wp-content/uploads/2023/10/02-BMS-ConsensusStatement-BMS-WHC-2020-Recommendations-on-HRT-in-menopausal-women-SEPT2023-A.pdf

REFERENCES

2   NHS UK (2023) Benefits and risks of hormone replacement therapy (HRT). www.nhs.uk/medicines/hormone-replacement-therapy-hrt/benefits-and-risks-of-hormone-replacement-therapy-hrt